Supported by the National Fund
for Academic Publication in Science and Technology

State of the Art in Long-Term Liver Cancer Survival

Breakthrough in Conception

Zengchen Ma, MD   **Qinghai Ye**, MD

Science Press
Beijing

Responsible Editor: Xiaoling Yang

Copyright © 2019 by Science Press.

Published by Science Press.

16 Donghuangchenggen North Street

Beijing 100717, China

Printed in Beijing.

ISBN 978-7-03-063544-0(Beijing)

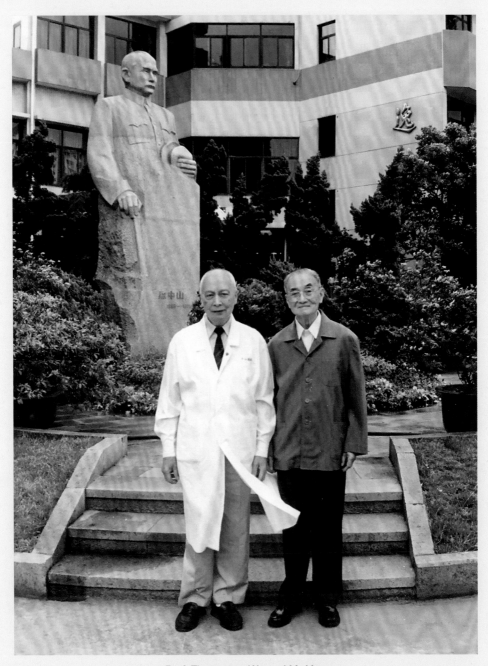

Prof. Zhaoguang Wu and Mr. Yang

43 years survival after resection for primary liver cancer in 1961.
Prof. Wu initiated resection of liver cancer at Zhongshan Hospital
and broke through the 40-year survival mark.
Photo taken in May 2000, at Zhongshan Hospital, Shanghai

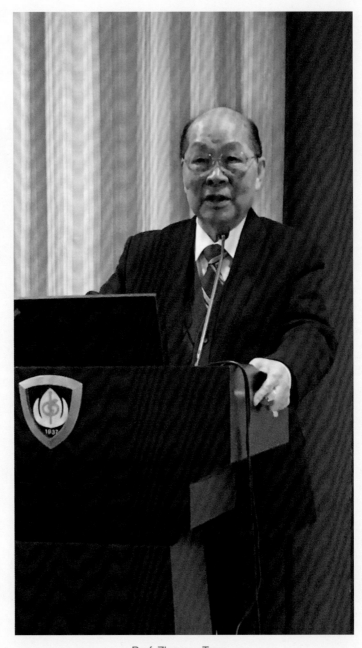

Prof. Zhaoyou Tang

Founder and Chairman of Liver Cancer Institute
Member of the Chinese Academy of Engineering
Pioneer in Small Liver Cancer Research
Photo taken in Mar 2019 at Zhongshan Hospital, Shanghai

State of the Art in Long-Term Liver Cancer Survival

Breakthrough in Conception

88 Cases 20–48 Years Survival

Science Press
Beijing

About the Author

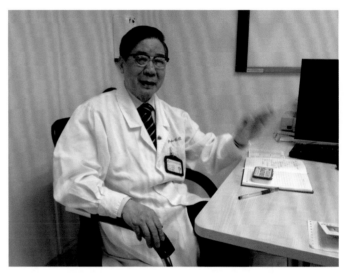

Photo taken at Zhongshan Hospital, Shanghai(Oct 2014)

Professor **Zengchen Ma** (1940–   ), Senior Oncology Surgeon and former Chief of Hepatic Surgery at Zhongshan Hospital (Fudan University), graduated from Faculty of Medicine, Beijing Medical University in 1965. He received the Master Degree in Hepatic Surgery from Shanghai First Medical University in 1981. He was also Visiting Scholar in Hepatic Surgery at Memorial Sloan-Kettering Cancer Center and Mount Sinai Medical Center, New York City from 1990–1991.

Prof. Ma has engaged in clinical practice and research at the Liver Cancer Institute, Zhongshan Hospital (Fudan University and former Shanghai First Medical University) for 40 years. Led by Prof. Zhaoyou Tang, MCAE, he is the principal researcher of several major scientific projects. His main contributions included, first national human liver cancer transplantation nude mice model (1982), first report of global longest survival for liver cancer (1993), predictive value of liver cirrhosis in AFP negative primary liver cancer (PLC, 1998), missed diagnosis of PLC with low level AFP (20–200µg/L) (2002) and initial statements on the three-stage radical resection standards for PLC (2004). His thesis on radical resection standards for PLC had been awarded the annual prestigious paper of *Chinese Journal of Oncology* and the 4th Outstanding Academic Works of the Chinese Association for

Science and Technology Journals (2005).

With over 40 years of surgical oncology experience, he not only excelled in diagnosis and treatment of liver cancer, but also performed clinical practice as an art. He took a patient-oriented and humanistic conception as guidance, emphasized pre-operative assessment instead of surgical indication, made decisions in the patient's benefit and not the treatment. Unlike the "Simple Removal Theory", he advocated combining resection, surgical risks and survival together, and acted as a pioneer in pursuing the long-term survival goal of over 10 years after hepatic surgery for decades.

His experiences included more than 2,000 cases of liver operation and 200 cases of resection for hepatic hilum lesions. He also succeeded in complicated resections of recurrence and repeated recurrence, two-step resection for cytoreduced liver cancer, resection of huge lesions with venous tumor thrombus, resection of secondary liver cancer and resection of liver cancer in a one and a half years old baby. He is the surgeon of a series of long-term PLC survivors, including over 100 cases more than 10 years and 40 cases more than 20 years. He always devoted himself to follow-up personally and experience documentation. As a serious observer, in May 2015, he witnessed an elderly patient with the longest longevity in the series survived 48 years after resection. He had published over 160 papers and co-edited the text *Practical Surgery of Hepatobiliary Tumors*. He was also the winner of the Shanghai Healthcare System 1991–1992 High Standard Medical Ethics Award.

About the Co-Author

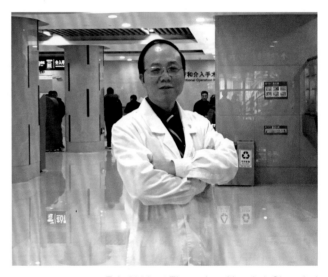

Feb 2019, at Zhongshan Hospital, Shanghai

Professor **Qinghai Ye** (1966–   ), Chief Physician/Tutor of Doctoral Graduate Students, Vice-Chief of Hepatic Surgery of Zhongshan Hospital (Fudan University), graduated from the Faculty of Medicine, Shanghai First Medical University in 1991 and received the Doctoral Degree in Hepatic Surgery from the Shanghai First Medical University in 1996. He is one of the Outstanding Talent of the Ministry of Education of the New Century, Shanghai Shuguang Project Scholar and Outstanding Academic Leader of Shanghai.

Since graduation, he has worked in the Dept. of Hepatic Surgical Oncology of Zhongshan Hospital for 27 years. He performs 500–600 hepatic tumor operations every year, including extended right hemi-hepatectomy, resection of hilar tumors and resection of the caudate lobe.

He has conducted the research of many important projects, such as the "973" National Basic Research Key Development Planning Project and Key Project of National Natural Science Foundation. He published more than 80 SCI articles, including in *Nature Medicine*, *Cancer Cell*, *Hepatology* and *Cancer Res*. He was awarded the Second Prize of National Natural Science, First Prize of Shanghai Natural Science and First Prize of Natural Science of the Ministry of Education.

Author

Zengchen Ma

Dept. of Surgical Hepatic Oncology, Zhongshan Hospital; Liver Cancer Institute, Fudan University, Shanghai, 200032 China

E-mail: mazengchen@me.com

Co-Author

Qinghai Ye

Dept. of Surgical Hepatic Oncology, Zhongshan Hospital; Liver Cancer Institute, Fudan University, Shanghai, 200032 China

E-mail: ye.qinghai@zs-hospital.sh.cn

Consultant

Zhaoyou Tang

Dept. of Surgical Hepatic Oncology, Zhongshan Hospital; Liver Cancer Institute, Fudan University, Shanghai, 200032 China

E-mail: zytang88@163.com

Zhaoguang Wu

Dept. of General Surgery, Zhongshan Hospital, Fudan University, Shanghai, 200032, China

E-mail: zgwu2000@163.com

Staff of Zhongshan Hospital Involved in Diagnosis and Treatment

Dept. of Surgical Hepatic Oncology

Zhaoyou Tang, Yeqin Yu, Xinda Zhou, Zengchen Ma, Zhiquan Wu, Jia Fan, Jian Zhou, Qinghai Ye, Shuangjian Qiu, Huichuan Sun, Yao Yu, Xiaowu Huang, Ning Ren, Yang Xu, Jian Sun, Xiaoying Huang, Yinghong Shi, Yongsheng Xiao, Pei Chen, Qiman Sun, Kang Song, Guoming Shi, Cheng Huang, Yifeng He, Zheng Wang, Yinghao Shen, Guohuang Yang, Zaozhuo Shen, Jianwen Cheng, Liuxiao Yang and Qiang Gao

Dept. of Medical Hepatic Oncology

Zhiying Lin, Jizhen Lu, Binghui Yang, Shenglong Ye, Yuhong Gan, Zhenggang Ren, Jinglin Xia, Yanhong Wang, Boheng Zhang, Ningling Ge, Yi Chen, Lixin Li, Fan Le, Rong Xin Chen and Biwei Yang

Liver Cancer Laboratory

Yinkun Liu, Kangda Liu, Zhuyuan Yu, Huizhi Weng, Weizhong Wu and Binbin Liu

Follow-up Unit of Liver Cancer Institute

Yueying Xu, Yuexiu Pan, Yu Zhang, Xiaomei Yang and Lijin Lu

Former Staff of Liver Cancer Institute

Yunzhen Cao, Nanqiao Zhou, Yanming Bao, Rong Yang, Min Zhou, Gang Zhao, Ming Zhang, Haiyan Zhou, Qi Ding, Dongbo Xu, Xiaomin Wang, Mingde Luo, Xuesheng Feng, Min Chen, Liwen Huang, Lunxiu Qin, Lu Wang, Lu Lu and Qi Pan

Fellows, Dept. of Surgical Hepatic Oncology

Shiguang Qian, Yu Xu, Xiaoyue Chen, Chunzhi Hao, Xingyao Huang, Jinqing Li, Shuzhou Chen, Weilun Yang, Shaoqin Zhao, Xusheng Li, Hongjie Sun, Renkuan Meng, Yongnan Hua, Zuojiang Liu, Shengqiu Wang, Yiren Zhao, Youzhi Han, Qunying Chen, Dagui Tong, Rudai Chen, Juzhou Zhang, Yun Hu, Liming Li, Cunshi Feng, Baoquan Jia, Zhifeng Li, Shouyuan Guo, Peile Huang, Weilun Yang, Zhenhou Yu, Te'er Ba, Maorong Li, Weiping Yang, Gang Huang, Chunyuan Du, Jiaqi Xu, Lianru Zhang, Nanwu Yang, Fahong Zheng, Qinyi Li, Huizhong Zhang, Jun He, Deting Zhan, Binghong Yu, Zimiao HU, Chenghong Wang, Jinbiao Gao, Yi Tang, Shiping Li, Jingen Zhang, Jiansheng Li, Xuecheng Wang, Yumin Zhou, Guangrong Cai, Jianhuai Zhang, Huandong Lin, Yuanzheng Wang, Guozhi Hu, Xiufang Zhu, Jinhui Xiong and Wei Zhang

Graduate Students and Interns of Dept. of Surgical Hepatic Oncology

Shuqun Cheng, Yaxin Zheng, Fangxian Sun, Qi Zhu, Lianhai Zhang, Rongxun Sun, Wen Qian, Yiqing Xu, Jia Bi, Ling Gong, Hong Ju and Hua Fan

Dept. of General Surgery

Youxian Feng, Zhaoguang Wu, Chengji Cai, Ronggui Zheng, Xianing Li, Guanghan Wu, Zhaohan Wu, Yibin Zhang, Weigang Xu, Liqing Yao, Yihong Sun, Weiqi Lu, Lujun Song and Yong Zhang

Dept. of Thoracic Surgery

Changyu Ren, Zhenbin Jiang, Zuyi Zhang, Yuanlin Shao and Qun Wang

Dept. of Vascular Surgery

Yuqi Wang

Dept. of Internal Medicine

Zhaoqi Lin, Meixian He, Naisheng Cai and Yuhong Zhou

Dept. of Anesthesia

Hao Jiang, Huizhen Pu, Fengying Lan, Zhanggang Xue, Yan Fang, Jing Cang, Zimin Su, Duming Zhu, Xiaoping Zhu and Yizhou He

Dept. of Diagnostic Radiology

Yingzhong Hong, Kangrong Zhou, Congde Xu, Zuwang Chen, Mengsu Zeng, Fuhua Yan, Yaping Jiang and Jiang Lin

Dept. of Ultrasound

Zhizhang Xu, Wenping Wang, Limin Liu, Beijian Huang, Hong Ding, Hui Zhang, Wanyuan He, Qing Qi and Zhengbiao Ji

Dept. of Interventional Radiology

Gui Lin, Xiaolin Wang, Jianhua Wang, Zhiping Yan and Jiemin Chen

Dept. of Pathology

Changchun Chen, Wensheng Pan, Yunshan Tan, Yingyong Hou and Yuan Ji

Dept. of Nuclear Medicine

Huiyang Zhao, Kejing Chen and Shaoliang Chen

Dept. of Radiotherapy

Zhaochong Zeng

Dept. of Traditional Chinese Medicine

Chenlong Tang

Dept. of Clinical Laboratory

Baishen Pan

Laboratory of Internal Medicine

Kang Zhou

Others Involved in Management

Dept. of Pathology, Former Shanghai First Medical University
Yueying Ying, Yuanding Xu, Weirong Zhai and Xiqi Hu

Shanghai Chest Hospital, Shanghai Jiaotong University
Yunzhong Zhou

Huashan Hospital, Fudan University
Quanxing Ni

Shanghai Tumor Hospital, Fudan University
Erxin Yu, Shouye Liu, Weiyu Tang, Yingqiang Shi

Children's Hospital, Fudan University
Xianmin Xiao

Huadong Hospital, Fudan University
Guozhen Zhang, Gensheng Wang, Yue Zhu

Shanghai Sixth People's Hospital, Shanghai Jiaotong University
Yongchang Zhou

Renji Hospital, Shanghai Jiaotong University
Encong Tang

Shanghai Rihui Hospital
Wuwu Luo, Zhenglai Zhou

Faculty of Medicine, Chinese University of Hong Kong
Liven Huang

Shanghai American-Sino Women and Children's Hospital
Haoping Zhu

Ganzhou People's Hospital, Jiangxi Province
Lianhui Zhang

Fuzhou Military General Hospital
Yi Jiang

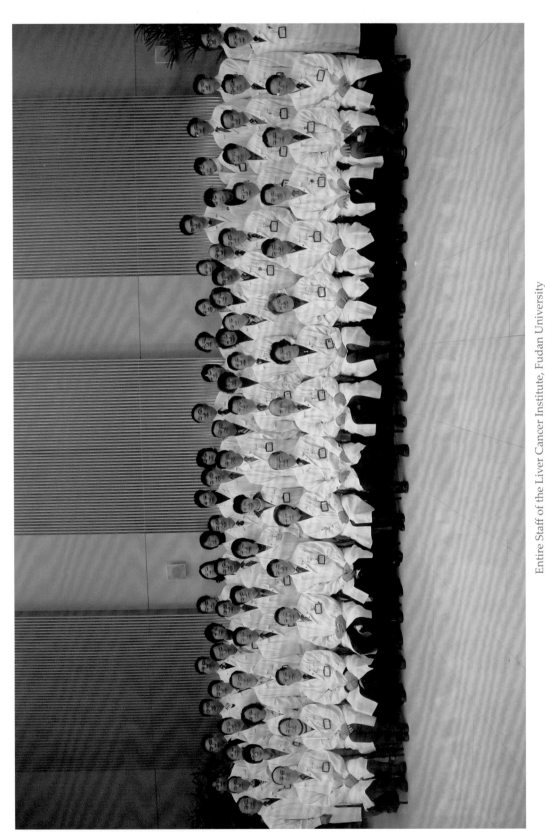

Entire Staff of the Liver Cancer Institute, Fudan University

Front row from right to left: Yinkun Liu, Zhenggang Ren, Jia Fan, Shenglong Ye, Chenlong Tang, Jizhen Lu, Xinda Zhou, Zhaoyou Tang (Chairman), Zhiying Lin, Zengchen Ma (Author), Zhiquan Wu, Kangda Lu, Binbin Liu, Huichuan Sun. Second row, right 8th: Qinghai Ye (Co-author) Dec 2009 at Zhongshan Hospital, Shanghai

Summary

This book introduces 20–48 years long-term survival after surgery in 88 liver cancer patients treated at Zhongshan Hospital during 1961 to 1995. The diagnosis of liver cancer was confirmed by pathology in all patients. One patient survived 43 years after resection in 1961. He was the first to breakthrough the 40 years survival mark after surgery. Another patient survived 48 years after only a single resection and is the longest survivor. The oldest patient is 99 years old living and well 40 years after liver resection and resection of subsequent pulmonary metastasis. The youngest patient is an $1^1/_2$-year-old child, who survived 22 years after resection. The first patient mentioned above died at the age of 93 and the other three are still alive and well. These successful cases indicate that liver cancer is treatable and at least in part curable, these results strongly strengthened our confidence in the battle against liver cancer. Meanwhile, the management of liver cancer is emphasized as a complex systematic project. One must strictly enforce regular follow-up and timely active treatment for recurrence or metastasis to achieve satisfactory results. The book consists of 8 parts that include brief history, treatment modalities, technological key points, successful experiences, knowledge of the connotation of liver cancer surgery, etc. The authors are witness or surgeon of the 88 cases. The book is written in plain language, with many photos, making it suitable for oncologists, hepatologists, gastroenterologists, general surgeons, primary care physicians, family physicians, young doctors, medical students, as well as all others with a common interest.

Preface

Liver cancer was considered an incurable disease in the past and the King of cancers. Life expectancy of patients was only 3–6 months after onset of symptoms. Presently, with advanced science and technology, it witnessed a breakthrough in diagnosis and treatment. The most prominent manifestation is extended survival of patients.

In the 1960s, clinical research in liver cancer was initiated at Zhongshan Hospital (affiliated to the former Shanghai First Medical College), Fudan University. The patient operated by Professor Zhaoguang Wu in 1961 survived for 43 years. Another patient operated by Professor Youxian Feng in 1967 is still alive with ongoing survival of 48 years. A patient resected in 1975 by Prof. Zhaoyou Tang (Member of Chinese Academy of Engineering) and Prof. Yeqin Yu at age 99, has a long-term ongoing survival of 40 years. With the advent of AFP, discovery of its relation with liver cancer and the implement of liver cancer screening in 1971, treatment results have significantly improved, especially after establishment of the Liver Cancer Institute at Zhongshan Hospital in 1969. By May 2015, 88 treated patients had survived 20 or more years. Such long-term survival has rarely been reported. It is a breakthrough in the clinical research of liver cancer that created a new dawn in treatment.

We report here the 88 cases subjected to surgery during 1961–1995, confirmed by pathology and with extended survival of 20 years or more. We participated or witnessed their surgery. Patients lost to follow-up, survival less than 20 years or data incomplete were not included.

Survival improved to a few months or even 1–3 years fail to reflect the latest progress in clinical research. Patients also are not contended to have just this amount of extension. Improvement of 5–10 years should be the goal in future studies. This is not fantasy but an obligation on the part of hepatologists. In other words, 10 or even 20 years survival and their percentage should be indispensable parameters to assess the level of clinical research.

Long-term survival is a battle between cancer and anticancer forces. The battle is a systematic process of prolonged duration. It involves the rich experiences of clinicians, tenacious persistence of patients and comprehensive hospital support. Case 42 with 28 years survival is a good example. Hepatic artery ligation with cannulation was first performed to reduce size of the tumor. It was then resected. Subsequent lung and mediastinum metastases were resected and radiofrequency ablation applied to a residual liver recurrence. In addition, Chinese medicine, Western medicine, irradiation were all involved in treatment. The patient is still alive with high quality of life. This would not have been possible without scientific thinking, good judgment, superb surgical skills, regular follow-up, appropriate comprehensive treatment when needed and adherence on the part of the patient. Though such a prolonged complicated treatment program is not necessary in every case, one should be prepared to fight a long lasting battle.

Diversity in the bionature of liver cancer has been recognized through accumulation of experience. Histogenetically, liver cancer can be hepatocellular, cholangiocellular or a combination of both. As the hepatocellular variety is most prevalent in China, discussion will be devoted to it. It has the specific feature of not spreading to hilar nodes. Hence, there is no need to clear those nodes in radical resection. Liver cancer can vary in differentiation, malignancy and invasiveness, but most often are moderately differentiated. It is prone to recur and metastasize, but not inevitable. Alpha-fetoprotein could be positive or negative. Tumor could be single or multiple. Growth could be rapid, slow or even stagnant at times. Blood supply could be rich or poor and tumor thrombi could be found in some. Its behavior could be fulminant or docile, vital or dormant. The same strategy might trigger different responses in different patients. Some of the specific biofeatures could change reversely after treatment, like AFP positive becomes negative and vice versa. Lung metastasis signified a late stage disease, but some could still be salvaged, even curable. However, nothing could be done when spread is massive. The above experience strengthened our confidence to carry on the research and resect recurrence or metastasis. A deeper understanding of the bionature of liver cancer with more correct judgment and appropriate treatment, a more satisfactory effective result would be achieved.

Breakthrough is to go beyond tradition, convention and past achievements into a new unknown world. In cancer treatment, it has to withstand the test of time. It is a process of from conception to practice and back to conception after being validated. Long-term survival of patients will speak for its efficacy and value. A genuine breakthrough is repeatable and applicable, not just a flash in the air.

This book has several special features. First, it is the first long-term survival of liver cancer patients reported in this format with rich factual contents. For each case, basic personal data, clinical course, surgical mode, tumor size and location, pathology and prognosis were documented in detail. Case 57 was the most complicated. The patient had 3 different cancers and went through 6 surgeries. The battle lasted 50 years before the patient became tumor free. Second, to some extent this monograph represents the latest state of art in the surgical treatment of liver cancer. Part Ⅵ "Hepatic Artery Procedure and the Two-step Resection for Liver Cancer" is an innovation extension of the traditional rationale of hepatic surgery. Third, the documented data are original works.

We have been working in the Dept. of Surgical Hepatic Oncology respectively for 40 and 27 years and are the surgeon-in-charge or surgeon of some of the 88 cases. We have witnessed the long-term survivals and done much of the registration, documentation, follow-ups, checkups, revisits and photography concerned. Most of these data have never been officially published before. Taking into account the large volume of cases, the long period of time, complicated treatment procedures as well as writing constraints and our limited knowledge, there might be ill considered and insufficient discussion, even errors in this book. We would be grateful and appreciative if readers could exchange ideas with us and point out our mistakes.

Zengchen Ma & Qinghai Ye

March 2019 in Shanghai

Contents

Part I

Eighty-Eight
Illustrative Cases

Liver cancer has long been known as a deadly disease with poor prognosis. Lifespan is short, counted in months even with treatment. This gloomy impression is imprinted deeply in the minds of the lay and professional. Liver surgery was nonexistent until first reported from Europe in the 1880s. However, its impact did not change this gloomy state. As liver cancer is very prevalent in China, Chinese clinicians took on the challenge to extend survival of this disease. Through years of dealing with this disease, we have encountered a different scenario. We have been able to witness long-term survival and not in just a few. Lifespan has been extended to be counted in years and no longer only in months. Reports began to appear like a spark of light in the dark that lighted up hope in our hearts. Hu and Wu reported 4 cases in 1979, Wang et al reported 5 cases in 1982 and Li was able to collect 89 cases from 16 institutions in 1988. Ma, Tang et al reported a much larger series of 113 cases in 2001. Ma, Wu reported in 2008 the longest survival of 43 years. Zhou et al reported 53 cases of over 20 years survival in 2009. We present herewith our meager successive experience to share with and hope to arouse the attention of those colleagues that have a mutual interest in this disease.

Our 88 cases had all been confirmed by surgery and pathology. Their clinical course had been documented in detail. The authors either witnessed or participated in their treatment. Case 1 resected in 1961 was the first to breakthrough the 40-year survival mark and case 2 operated in 1967 had the longest ongoing survival of 48 years. Case 69 was the youngest patient one and a half years old, with ongoing survival of 22 years. The oldest patient, case 12 operated in 1975 at age 60 was 99 and in good health on follow-up in 2015. Many of our patients were complicated and difficult cases. Our results tend to tell us that liver cancer is treatable and may even be curable. Surgical resection and followed by comprehensive treatment when indicated will salvage patients and afford them a long-term good quality of life is beyond any doubt.

Case 1

(Admission No. 35874)

Recurrence 39 Years after Resection, Total Survival 43 Years

(Nov. 1961–Jan. 2005)

Synopsis

Mr. Yang, bank clerk, was born in Shanghai, China. Diagnosis of primary liver cancer was confirmed by surgery and pathology. He came to Zhongshan Hospital because he palpated a movable mass in the left hypochondrium. Laboratory investigation was essentially normal. GI series showed the mass was intimately related to the lesser curvature of the stomach. In Nov 1961 at age 50, he underwent laparotomy under ether general anesthesia. Dr. Zhaoguang Wu was the surgeon. A 10cm huge tumor with clear margin originated from the undersurface of the left lateral lobe of the liver and indented deeply on the lesser curvature of the stomach. The liver was normal otherwise. Partial resection of the left lateral lobe was carried out without any difficulty. Pathologic diagnosis was hepatocellular carcinoma (HCC) with no liver cirrhosis. Recovery was smooth and he was discharged on day 9. He resumed work at one and a half months and lived a healthy, normal life. He received regular follow-up at the Dept. of Surgical Hepatic Oncology. In the 39th post-op year, Dec 1999, at age 89, 2 recurrent tumors were found on type-B ultrasound and CT scanning. His AFP from negative gradually became positive and maximally reached 60,500μg/L. As his general condition was frail with compromised cardiopulmonary functions, surgery was not considered. Percutaneous ethanol injections and microwave ablation were carried out by the Dept. of Ultrasound and Dept. of Medical Hepatic Oncology with eradication of the recurrence in the left lateral lobe. He lived another 5 years with residual cancer in the left medial lobe, but died of cardiopulmonary failure in Jan 2005, at age 93, with a disease-free survival of 38 years and overall survival of 43 years.

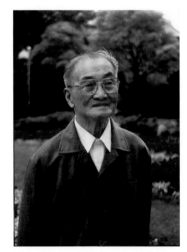

Fig. 1.1   Total 43 years survival after resection of liver cancer in Nov 1961 at age 50 and died in Jan 2005 at age 93. Photo taken in May 2000 at Zhongshan Hospital, by Aini Lin

Other Relevant Data

Aside from his mother died of liver cancer, there was no other history of any liver disease in the family. At present, liver cancer can be divided into AFP-positive and AFP-negative. In the early days when Mr. Yang came to the hospital, AFP was not yet available. However, judging from his high AFP (60,500µg/L) at recurrence, he presumably belonged to the AFP-positive group.

Surgeon's Profile

Prof. Zhaoguang Wu, senior general surgeon, was born 1925 in Beijing, China. He was former Chief of General Surgery, Zhongshan Hospital, Shanghai First Medical College (his Alma Mater). In 1949 he went to the US for surgical training, returned in 1956 and joined the Dept. of Surgery of Shanghai Zhongshan Hospital. In 1957, he carried out a right hepatic trisectionectomy for gallbladder cancer. Subsequently, he also performed successfully a left trisectionectomy for liver cancer with a subcostal incision in the early 1960s. In Nov 1961, he operated on Mr. Yang, who survived 43 years and became the first to breakthrough the 40-year survival mark after surgery.

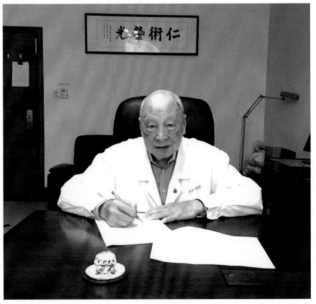

Fig. 1.2   Prof. Zhaoguang Wu, surgeon of the liver resection (Dec 2016)

Among his many achievements, the following could be outstanding. The scenario is a 27 years old female who lost her entire jejunum, ileum, ascending colon and right half transverse colon because of volvulus of her small bowel. The duodenum was directly connected to the left half of her transverse colon. She was put on Total Parenteral Nutrition, progressed to Home Parenteral Nutrition and led a normal life for 30 years (Feb 1986 to Jun 2016). She gave birth to a girl in Apr 1992. This daughter is now a college graduate and mother of a newborn girl.

Background

In the 1960s, regarding liver cancer both clinical experience and research were limited. AFP was not only unavailable, imaging equipment was very meager and simple with only type-A ultrasound and isotope liver scanning. Diagnostic accuracy and sensitivity were low. Laparotomy was often performed for diagnosis and treatment. This patient directly underwent exploration because of the palpable abdominal mass.

Though general and epidural anesthesia are widely applied nowadays, they were not yet fully introduced in the1960s. Mr Yang's

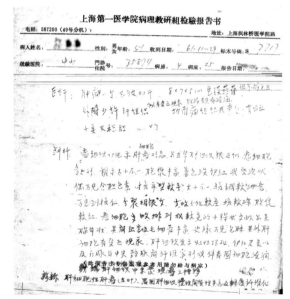

Fig. 1.3   Pathology report of resected specimen: Hepatocellular carcinoma

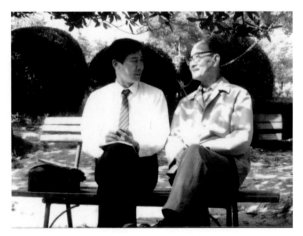

Fig. 1.4   Patient on follow-up with Dr. Ma (left) of the Liver Cancer Institute (May 1990)

operation was performed under open mask ether general anesthesia.

Though the general utility midline vertical incision affords rapid access to abdominal visceral organs with minimal trauma, it is not conducive to thoroughly mobilize ligaments around the liver and expose a deep-seated tumor of the liver, unless extended unusually in length. Nowadays, the subcostal incision is the gold standard of optimal approach for hepatic surgery.

Discussion

The good therapeutic effect of 38 years tumor-free existence is probably because the tumor is of only low grade malignancy and resection relatively thorough. In addition, there might be some relationship with his stable mental status, positive personality and healthy life style. He always took a peaceful and patient attitude regarding illness and life. He actively cooperated with his attending physicians, led a regulated life and lived on balanced nutrition without unusual dietary habits.

Unfortunately, the tumor recurred after 39 years, denoting refractoriness of the cancer. Once a patient's immune system became compromised, the residual dormant cancer cells would come out of "hibernation". Therefore, even after a curative resection, one should never be blindly optimistic and ignore regular follow-up. He was tumor-free for 38 years, cancer recurred in the 39th post-op year. This implies that it is mandatory every liver cancer patient should be followed for life.

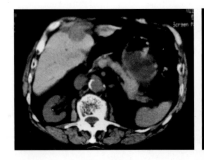 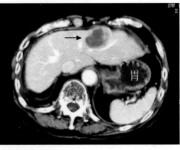 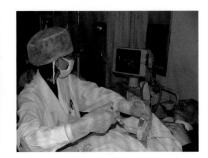

Fig. 1.5   Left: Two recurrent tumors In the 39th post-op year on B-US and CT scanning (Nov 2000); Right: Residual recurrence in the left medial lobe (Nov 2001)

Fig. 1.6   Ultrasound guided percutaneous ethanol injection for recurrence (May 2003)

Even though he had residual cancer when he died, he was tumor-free for 38 years. As a whole, he lived for over 40 years with acceptable quality of life. He could be considered a successful case of liver cancer resection.

Moreover, he was the first patient to have a recurrence 38 years after resection.

Key Points to Remember

Mr. Yang was the first patient to survive over 40 years after liver cancer resection in China. He was the first to reach over 90 years old as a liver cancer patient. Moreover, he was also the first to have a recurrence 38 years after resection.

Case 2

(Admission No. 75843)
A Single Resection, Ongoing Survival 48 Years
(Nov 1967－)

Synopsis

Ms. Shi, teacher, was born Oct 1931, in Zhangjiagang, Jiangsu, China. Diagnosis of primary liver cancer was confirmed by surgery and pathology. In Oct 1967, she came to Zhongshan Hospital, because of a palpable upper abdominal mass. On type-A ultrasound imaging, she was suspected to have primary liver cancer. In Nov 1967, she underwent exploration. Dr. Youxian Feng presided over her operation. A tumor, 6.5cm located in the left medial lobe (segment IV) and a left hemi-hepatectomy was carried out. Pathologic diagnosis was HCC. Postoperative recovery was smooth and no adjuvant treatment given. Follow-up by Nov 2015 at age 84, she was well with an ongoing tumor-free survival of 48 years.

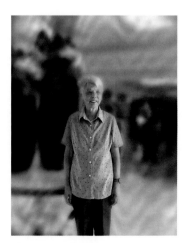

Fig. 1.7 Patient, 48 years ongoing survival after liver resection. Photo taken in Aug 2014

Other Relevant Data

Ms. Shi was healthy before being diagnosed to have liver cancer and she did not have any hepatic disease background.

In the 1960s, AFP, type-B ultrasound and CT scanning were not yet available. Her diagnosis depended mainly on type-A ultrasound.

No adjuvant therapy was given after operation.

The patient had a cheerful personality and was very sociable.

She had a wide-range of food options without any restrictions or unusual dietary whims.

Surgeon's Profile

Prof. Youxian Feng (1919–2008), senior surgeon, was born in Zhejiang, China. He was the former Chief of General Surgery and later Head of Vascular Surgery Unit at Zhongshan Hospital. He graduated from Shanghai Medical College in 1946. In Nov. 1967, he operated on Ms. Shi, who ongoing survived 48 years, the longest survivor after single resection of liver cancer.

Key Points to Remember

It is well known that liver cancer is prone to recur and metastasize. In

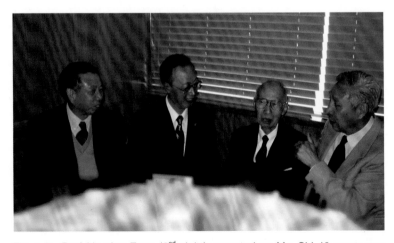

Fig. 1.8   Prof. Youxian Feng (2nd, right) operated on Ms. Shi 48 years ago, being visited by former colleagues on his 90th birthday in Oct 2008. Photo provided by Yuqi Wang (2nd, left), vascular surgeon and Director of Zhongshan Hospital

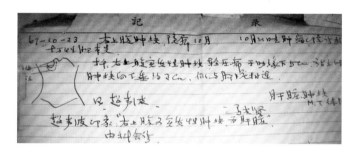

Fig. 1.9   Outpatient record by Prof. Youxian Feng who first attended the patient in 1967

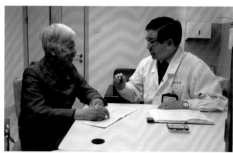

Fig. 1.10   Patient on regular post-op check-up. Photo taken In Nov 2014, the 47th post-op year

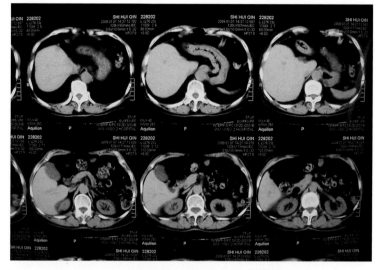

Fig. 1.11   CT (2009) showing no recurrence in the liver

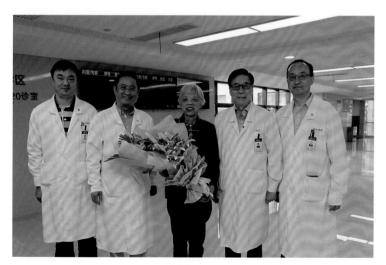

Fig. 1.12   Liver surgeons of Zhongshan Hospital congratulating patient on her health and longevity (Oct 2017)

reality, it is not inevitably so in every single case without exception. It can be surmised that her tumor had an inactive biologic character. On this basis, timely and thorough radical resection eventually led to an ideal effect. To obtain a good curative effect，the two above conditions are indispensable.

She was the longest survivor (48 years) of liver cancer in Zhongshan Hospital, and also the longest survivor with relatively complete data documented.

Case 3

(Admission No. 97713)
Two Resections, Total Survival 44 Years
(Jun 1968–Oct 2012)

Synopsis

Mr. Liao, educator, was born in Jiangxi, China. In June 1968, because of ruptured liver cancer he was explored by Dr. Lianhui Zhang in Ganzhou, Jiangxi. The 4cm tumor was located in the left lobe of the liver. A partial resection of the left liver was carried out. Pathology diagnosis was HCC. In Apr 1971, he was admitted to Zhongshan Hospital due to recurrence on isotope liver scanning. Dr. Tang presided over the 2nd operation and a left lateral lobectomy was performed. Recovery was smooth and no adjuvant therapy administered.

There was no recurrence or metastatic spread on follow-up. Unfortunately, in Oct 2012 at age 82, he died of uncontrolled bleeding from bladder cancer at his hometown. Nevertheless, he could be considered a successful case of liver cancer treated simply by surgery with 44 years survival.

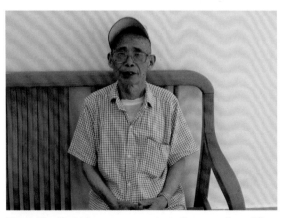

Fig. 1.13　Forty-four years survival after resection of liver cancer. Photo taken in Jun 2012 at Zhongshan Hospital

Surgeon's Profile

Prof. Zhaoyou Tang, was born Dec 1930 in Guangdong, China, a senior surgeon of Hepatic Oncology, founder of small liver cancer research, Chairman of Liver Cancer Institute of Fudan University (former Liver Cancer Institute of Shanghai First Medical University), Member of the Chinese Academy of Engineering and Vice Chairman of Oncology Society of CMA. He graduated from Shanghai First Medical College in 1954 and became a surgeon at Zhongshan Hospital.

Dr. Tang has devoted his life to research in hepatocellular carcinoma for more than 40 years. He won a Gold Medal Award from the Cancer Research Institute, New York, USA in 1979 and twice (1985 and 2006) the National First Prize Award for Progress in Science and Technology, P.R. China.

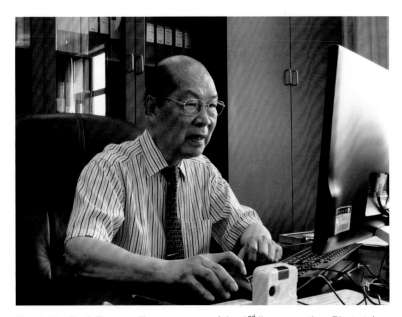

Fig. 1.14   Prof. Zhaoyou Tang, surgeon of the 2nd liver resection. Photo taken Aug 2015, age 85 at Zhongshan Hospital

Key Points to Remember

Prior to 1971, AFP assay and advanced imaging equipments were not yet available, a palpable abdominal mass and rupture of liver cancer were not necessarily a bad thing. These often urged the patient to timely

11

seek diagnosis and prompt treatment.

Although liver cancer and cirrhosis are the main causes of death in liver cancer, other morbidities such as malignant tumor in other organs, cerebral infarction, heart disease, accidents, etc could also lead to death. Therefore, longevity of a liver cancer patient depends not only on liver cancer therapeutic effect per se.

Case 4

(Admission No. 84147)
A Single Resection, Total Survival 26 Years
(Feb 1969–May 1995)

Synopsis

Mr. Bian, teacher was treated in Shanghai for an acute abdomen in Nov 1968. Operation found a liver cancer with rupture and bleeding. The tumor was not resected but bleeding controlled. Three months later, in Feb 1969 at age 40, he came to Zhongshang Hospital and underwent the 2nd operation. Dr Zhaoguang Wu presided over the procedure. A 3.5cm tumor was located in the left medial lobe of the liver. A regular left hemihepatectomy was carried out. Pathology report was HCC. Recovery was smooth and no adjuvant therapy given. Unfortunately, in May 1995 at age 66, he died of recurrence due to neglect of regular follow-up with 26 years survival.

Key Points to Remember

According to our experience, even very early liver cancer or very thorough resection cannot guarantee no recurrence. We believe that liver cancer patients should be followed life-long.

Furthermore, rupture of the cancer does not necessarily imply dissemination of the disease with no chance of being salvaged.

Case 5

(Admission No. 93987)
A Single Resection, Total Survival 34 Years
(Sep 1970–Sep 2004)

Synopsis

Mr. Zheng was born in Pinghu, Zhejiang, China. In Sep 1970 at age 58, he underwent liver cancer resection. A 9cm tumor located in the right lobe and a right hemihepatectomy with cholecystectomy was performed through a thoracoabdominal incision by Dr. Ronggui Zheng. Pathology report was HCC. Recovery and therapeutic results were satisfactory. There was no recurrence or metastasis on follow-up. In Sep 2004 at age 92, he died peacefully from old age with tumor-free survival of 34 years.

Discussion

In 1970s, due to inadequate equipment and experience, a thoracoabdominal incision was often used for right lobe liver resection. With advance in science and technology nowadays, a thoracoabdominal incision is no longer needed, regardless how complicated and difficult a right lobe resection.

Key Points to Remember

This case tells us that liver cancer is not necessarily highly malignant. Timely and thorough treatment with surgery is very effective. Long-term and even lifelong disease-free survival could be expected.

This is the 2nd patient age over 90 in this series.

Conclusion: Liver cancer patients can also enjoy longevity after thorough treatment.

Case 6

(Admission No. 98239)
A Single Resection of Giant Liver Cancer, Ongoing Survival
44 Years
(Aug 1971–Sep 2015)

Synopsis

Mr. Ma, farmer, was born in Yancheng, Jiangsu, China. In Aug 1971 at age 31, because of a palpable upper abdominal mass he was admitted to ZhangShan Hospital for exploration. Dr. Xianing Li presided over the operation. The 17cm tumor located in the left lobe of the liver. A left hemihepatectomy was carried out. The resected tumor weighted 1,050gm. Pathology report was HCC. Except for wound infection, post-op recovery was essentially smooth and no adjuvant therapy given. Follow-up by Sep 2015 at age 75, he was living and well with ongoing survival of 44years.

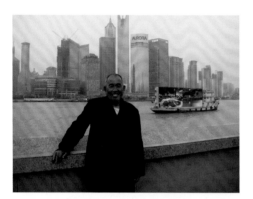

Fig. 1.15   Patient, 44 years ongoing survival after liver resection. Photo taken at the Bund, Shanghai in May 2008

Key Points to Remember

Huge and even giant (very huge) liver cancer is not a surgical contraindication. Part of them can have a good result. Even "a single resection can be once for all" like Mr. Ma. However, not all huge liver cancers are suitable for surgery. Operation in an advanced huge tumor is not only ineffective, but also harmful. Generally, advanced huge liver cancer usually has multiple satellite nodules or cancer thrombus in the portal trunk. For giant liver cancer but not advanced, we can carry out transcatheter arterial chemoembolization (TACE) or hepatic artery surgery (ligation, catheterization and intra-arterial chemotherapy) first, then perform a 2-step resection of the volume reduced tumor.

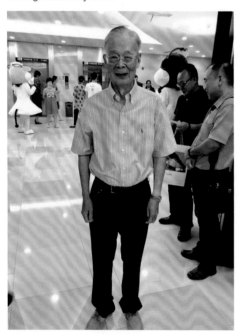

Fig. 1.16   Dr. Xianing Li, surgeon of the liver resection（Sep 2017）

Case 7

(Admission No. 106499)
A Single Resection, Total Survival 20 Years
(Mar 1973–Jul 1993)

Synopsis

Ms. Huang was born in Jiangsu, China. She came to ZhongShan Hospital because of right shoulder and right upper abdominal pain, positive AFP and a solid space-occupying lesion in the liver on isotope liver scanning. Diagnosis was liver cancer. In Mar 1973 at age 20, Dr. Zhaoyou Tang presided over the procedure. A 15cm well-defined huge tumor occupied almost the whole right liver. There was no satellite nodule or tumor thrombus. Right hemihepatectomy with cholecystectomy was performed. Pathology diagnosis was HCC. Recovery was smooth and no adjuvant therapy given. For 20 years she lived well. Unfortunately, in Jul 1993 at age 40, she died of recurrence due to neglect of regular follow-up and timely treatment.

Key Points to Remember

In 1973, AFP became available for diagnosis of primary liver cancer. This was the first patient identified as HCC on elevated AFP with positive isotope liver scanning in our series. Our experience is that positive AFP and a solid space-occupying lesion in the liver basically denote HCC. The other value of AFP is to monitor thoroughness of the resection. AFP in this patient dropped from 8,500µg/L to normal after resection. This could truly be called a radical resection.

This case once again showed that huge and even giant (very huge) liver cancer is not a contraindication to surgery. Part of them could be salvaged with relatively good results.

Case 8

(Admission No. 117455)
Liver Resection and Resection of Pulmonary Metastasis, Total Survival 32 Years
(Apr 1975–Apr 2007)

Synopsis

Mr. Chen, electrician, was born in Jiangsu, China and worked in Shanghai. He was admitted to Zhongshan Hospital because of a palpable upper abdominal mass, elevated AFP and a space-occupying lesion on isotope liver scanning. In Apr 1975 at age 45, he was explored by Dr Yeqin Yu. The 8cm tumor located in the left lateral lobe with tumor thrombus in the left hepatic vein and extended into the inferior vena cava was found. A left hemihepatectomy with removal of the tumor thrombus intact and *in toto* was performed. Convalescence was uneventful. Three years later, chest X-ray showed a 6cm suspicious metastatic lesion at the upper pole of the right lung. In Dec 1978, the 2nd operation right upper lobectomy of the lung was performed by Dr. Zhenbin Jiang. Pathology report of the lung specimen was HCC. After the 2nd operation, therapeutic outcome was basically satisfactory with tumor-free survival of 32 years. Unfortunately, in Apr 2007 at age 77, he died of progressive liver failure due to cirrhosis.

Other Relevant Data

This patient and family had no hepatic disease background. He was AFP positive, which dropped from 2,000µg/L and 1,000µg/L respectively to normal after the 2 resections.

Key Points to Remember

This is the 1st long-term survivor after resection of liver cancer and tumor thrombus removal. We feel that En Bloc resection should be advocated when liver cancer is accompanied by a tumor thrombus that can be easily and completely removed.

This is the first patient that survived more than 20 years after liver and metachronous pulmonary metastasis resections. As witnessed by this case, our experience substantially supported our unorthodox belief that lung metastasis does not necessarily warrant a death sentence. Actually, active and aggressive treatment can, in some instances, improve outcome favorably to a fairly satisfactory degree, even in patients with moderately advanced disease.

Case 9

(Admission No. 117983)
Two Resections, Ongoing Survival 40 Years
(Jun1975-   )

Synopsis

Mr. Chen was born in Shanghai, China. He was suspected to have liver cancer and admitted to Zhongshan Hospital due to elevated AFP during liver cancer screening. In Jun 1975 at age 30, he was explored by Dr Yeqin Yu. A 1.5cm tumor located in the left lateral lobe and a left lateral segmentectomy was performed. For 16 years, he lived well. In Sep 1991 at age 46, he was operated again by Dr. Yu for recurrence. The tumor was 4.5cm, located in the right posterior lobe. A partial hepatectomy was performed. Pathology was HCC. Follow-up by Sep 2015 at age 70, he was alive and well with ongoing 40 years survival.

Other Relevant Data

This patient and family had no hepatic disease background. His pre-op AFP levels were 350μg/L and 32μg/L respectively and both dropped to normal after resection.

Key Points to Remember

In liver cancer, recurrence or metastasis after surgery is not rare and even frequent. If we deal with recurrence and metastasis with a positive attitude and good technology, at times could yield good results and even create miracles. This is the second patient that survived another 20 years or more after his 2nd operation, with a total ongoing survival of 40 years or more in our series. We firmly believe resection for recurrence is an important way to improve the long-term curative effect.

Case 10

(Admission No. 119474)
Liver Resection and Resection of Pulmonary Metastasis, Total Survival 25 Years
(Aug 1975–Mar 2000)

Synopsis

Mr. Hu was born in Shanghai, China. He was admitted to Zhongshan Hospital because of elevated AFP during liver cancer screening and a space-occupying lesion on isotope liver scanning. In Aug 1975 at age 42, he was explored by Dr Yeqin Yu. The 3cm tumor located in the left medial lobe of the liver close to the gallbladder and a left hemihepatectomy with cholecystectomy was performed. Pathology was HCC. Three years later, his AFP rose again, hepatic arteriography ruled out recurrence in the liver. A chest film showed a 2cm suspicious metastatic lesion in the middle lobe of the right lung. In May 1978 at age 45, a right middle lobectomy of the lung was performed by Dr. Zhenbin Jiang. Pathology of the lung specimen was metastatic HCC. Unfortunately, in Mar 2000 at age 67, he died of recurrence with a total survival of 25 years.

Other Relevant Data

This patient was AFP-positive which dropped from 320µg/L and 150µg/

L respectively to normal after the resections.

Key Points to Remember

This is the 2nd patient that survived more than 20 years after liver and metachronous pulmonary metastasis resections. Unfortunately, he neglected regular follow-ups and lost the opportunity for further timely treatment and ongoing survival.

Case 11

(Admission No. 118533)
A Single Resection, Ongoing Survival 40 Years
(Jul 1975-   )

Synopsis

Mr. Qin was born in Shanghai, China. In Dec 1974, AFP was positive during liver cancer screening and continued to rise to 4,500μg/L on observation. Although type-A ultrasound and isotope liver scanning were both negative, primary liver cancer was highly suspected. In Jun 1975 at age 21, he was explored with consent. The 3cm tumor located in the right lower part of the liver and a partial liver resection was performed by Dr. Yeqin Yu. Pathology was HCC. Follow-up by Sep 2015 at age 61, there was no recurrence or metastasis. He is another typical "a simple resection can be once for all" case with ongoing survival of 40 years.

Other Relevant Data

This patient and family had no hepatic disease background. His AFP dropped from 4,500μg/L to normal after resection.

Key Points to Remember

Usually, diagnosis of liver cancer relies mainly on imaging which is important for performing surgery. As a rule, a patient suspected of HCC but not confirmed by imaging, such as type-B ultrasound, CT or MRI is not considered for surgery. In the early 1970s, this patient was explored because no advanced sensitive imaging equipment was available at that time, and a high AFP strongly suggested HCC. Courage on the part of the surgeon was essential and commendable. On the other hand, the patient consented to have surgery was also important.

Case 12

(Admission No. 119731)
Oldest Survivor, Age 99, after Liver Resection and Subsequent Pulmonary Metastasis Resection, Ongoing Survival 40 Years
(Sep 1975–)

Synopsis

Mr. Shen was born in Chongming, Shanghai, China. He came to Zhongshan Hospital because of a palpable upper abdominal mass, elevated AFP and a space occupying lesion on isotope liver scanning. He underwent 2 operations. In Sep 1975 at age 60 Dr. Zhaoyou Tang and Dr. Yeqin Yu performed the 1st operation. The isolated huge 12cm tumor was located in the left lateral lobe. A left hemihepatectomy was performed. Four years later, a 5cm metastatic lesion, in the left upper lobe of the lung was found. In Oct 1979 a left upper lobectomy of the lung was performed by Dr. Changyu Ren. Pathology of the lung specimen was HCC. Follow-up by Oct 2015, the patient was 99 years old with ongoing tumor-free survival of 40 years.

Other Relevant Data

This patient and family had no hepatic disease background. He had elevated AFP which dropped from 1,500μg/L and 30μg/L respectively

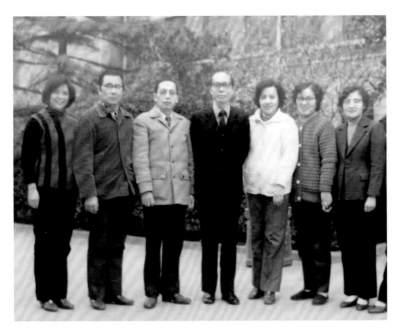

Fig. 1.17   Part of medical team of 40 years ongoing survival after liver resection and subsequent pulmonary metastasis resection. Surgeons of the liver resection: Dr. Zhaoyou Tang (middle), Dr. Yeqin Yu (3rd, left). Photo taken in Dec 1986 at Zhongshan Hospital

to normal after the 2 resections.

He underwent a subtotal gastrectomy for ulcer bleeding in Yunnan in 1976 and had a mild cerebral infarction, but with treatment recovered uneventfully.

His secret of keeping healthy after major operations could be summarized as: a result of correctly accepted the impact of being ill, actively collaborated with his medical team, and maintained a balanced, optimistic and cheerful mental state. Moreover, he had a wide-range of food options, including chicken and sea food without any unusual dietary habits.

Key Points to Remember

Normally, life expectancy meeting or exceeding the 100-year mark is rare, especially when inflicted with cancer. Mr. Shen, age 99, created a record of being the oldest patient alive after resection of liver cancer.

This was the 3rd patient over 20 years long-term survival after liver resection and resection of subsequent pulmonary metastasis. He was the oldest and also the longest survivor (36 years) of the 3 patients that had liver and subsequent lung resection. Our experience is that lung metastasis after liver cancer resection is not necessarily surgically contraindicated and long-term survival after radical resection of metastasis could be expected in some patients.

Case 13

(Admission No. 119619)
A Single Resection, Ongoing Survival 40 Years
(Sep 1975⁻)

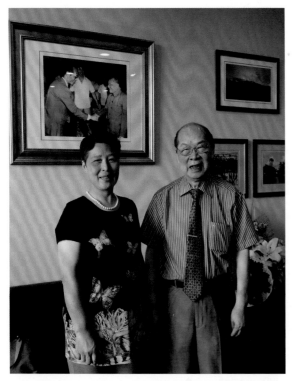

Fig. 1.18   Patient, 40 years ongoing survival after a single resection of liver cancer. Prof. Zhaoyou Tang (surgeon) and patient (left). Sep 2015 at Zhongshan Hospital

Synopsis

Ms. Pan was born in Shanghai, China. She came to Zhongshan Hospital because of elevated AFP 4,500μg/L during liver cancer screening. At that time, advanced imaging examinations were not available. Nevertheless, liver cancer was still highly suspected. In Sep 1975 at age 20, she consented to be explored. A 4cm tumor located in the left lateral lobe of the liver and a left hemihepatectomy was performed by Dr Zhaoyou Tang and Dr. Yeqin Yu. Pathology report was HCC. Follow-up by Sep 2015 at age 59, she was healthy with ongoing tumor-free 40 years survival.

Other Relevant Data

This patient had a history of hepatitis but no family history of liver cancer.

Her AFP dropped from 4,500μg/L to normal after surgery.

Except taking Chinese herbal medicine for a year, no other adjuvant therapy was employed.

Her personality was cheerful, optimistic, willing to share her cancer experience and transfer positive attitudes to benefit fellow patients.

She led a well regulated life, paying attention to work and rest. She also had a wide-range of food options with no unusual dietary whims.

She married in 1985 and accepted the advice "not to have a child too early", within 10 years of surgery. The next year, she gave birth to a healthy baby girl. Her daughter has now graduated from college and has a job to her liking.

Key Points to Remember

There is no unanimous consensus whether patients can have children after operation for liver cancer. Because liver cancer is prone to recur and metastasize, especially in the early post-op period, our tentative opinion is that they should delay gestation for at least 5 years.

Case 14

(Admission No. 136383)
A Single Resection, Total Survival 31 Years
(May 1978–Sep 2009)

Synopsis

Mr. Zhou was born in Jiangsu, China. His AFP was elevated during liver cancer screening. Hepatic arteriogram showed a suspicious cancer lesion. In May 1978 at age 38, he was explored. The tumor 1.5cm was located in the right lobe close to the gallbladder. A partial liver resection with cholecystectomy was performed by Dr. Zhaoyou Tang and Xinda Zhou. Pathology report was HCC. Recovery was smooth and no adjuvant therapy given. Unfortunately, 27 years later, his cancer recurred. Treatment with Traditional Chinese Medicine the only option then for 4 years failed to control the disease. In Sep 2009 at age 69, he died with a total survival of 31 years.

Key Points to Remember

Long-term survival is not only determined by stage of the disease and thoroughness of resection, it also depended on whether recurrence is detected early, intensity and timeliness of the needed treatment. Usually, it is easier said than done. However, regular follow-up, early detection and surgical treatment are of paramount importance.

Case 15

(Admission No. 138695)
A Single Resection, Total Survival 34 Years
(Sep 1978–May 2013)

Synopsis

Mr. Wang was born in Shanghai, China. He had elevated AFP during liver cancer screening and a space-occupying lesion in the right liver on isotope liver scanning. In Sep 1978 at age 43, he was explored. The 7cm tumor located in the lower part of the right liver and a partial liver resection was performed by Dr. Yeqin Yu and Dr. Xinda Zhou. Pathology report was HCC. His AFP dropped from 2,000μg/L to normal. Unfortunately, after more than 30 years, due to neglect of regular follow-up, when recurrence was detected, it was already too advanced and beyond possible salvage. In May 2013 at age 78, he died with a total survival of 34 years.

Key Points to Remember

In the early 1970s, liver cancer was usually not easily found early, because patients often were asymptomatic and sophisticated diagnostic equipment not available. The advent of AFP screening is beneficial in early detection and early treatment. Mr. Wang was harvested through screening. As he was detected early and treated timely yielded a good outcome. At that time, screening with AFP was of positive significance. It salvaged many patients and promoted in-depth development in liver cancer research.

However, the cost of mass survey is prohibitive, not suitable for large-scale promotion.

This is the 3rd case of over 30 years survival but finally died of recurrence. It tells us, that no matter how long survival is, follow-up should never be ignored.

Case 16

(Admission No. 138457)
A Single Resection, Ongoing Survival 36 Years
(Nov 1978-　)

Synopsis

Mr. Jin was born in Shanghai, China. His AFP was elevated during liver cancer survey in Apr 1978, but type-A ultrasound imaging was not relevant. As he felt fit and well, surgery was refused. AFP persistently remained elevated. He finally consented to be explored. In Nov 1978 at age 24, a 3cm tumor located in segments Ⅱ - Ⅲ of the liver was found and a left lateral lobectomy was performed by Dr. Yeqin Yu and Dr. Xinda Zhou. Pathology report was moderately differentiated HCC with cirrhosis. Recovery was uneventful. No specific adjuvant therapy was employed and therapeutic result satisfactory. His AFP dropped from 340μg/L to normal. Follow-up by Sep 2015 at age 60, he was healthy with ongoing survival of 36 years.

Key Points to Remember

This is another successful case diagnosed by AFP alone without confirmation on imaging studies. Operation ultimately achieved long-term survival. With the advent of sophisticated diagnostic equipment, the above situation is very rare. At present, we do not advocate abdominal exploration blindly.

This is another case with long-term survival. It tells us that early curative resection plays a key role in the treatment of liver cancer.

Case 17

(Admission No. 140030)
A Single Resection, Total Survival 25 Years
(Dec 1978–Apr 2003)

Synopsis

Mr. Zhang, technician, born in Shanghai, China, was AFP positive on liver cancer survey. Isotope liver scanning showed a space-occupying lesion in the liver. In Dec 1978 at age 48, he was explored. The 3.7cm tumor located in the right lobe and a partial hepatectomy was performed by Dr. Yeqing Yu and Dr. Xinda Zhou. Pathology report was HCC. AFP dropped from 18,000μg/L to normal. Unfortunately, in Apr 2003 at age 73, he was killed in a traffic accident with total survival of 25 years.

Key Points to Remember

Recurrence and metastasis of liver cancer can lead to death. Other malignancies, cardiovascular diseases, cerebrovascular accidents as well as natural and man-made disasters could also lead to death. Therefore, long-term survival and longevity of patients depend not only on curative effect of the cancer treatment, but also whether serious comorbidities or lethal accidents exist. In this case, Mr. Zhang was a victim of a traffic accident that ended his precious life. His survival was cut short to 25 years.

Case 18

(Admission No. 140470)
A Single Resection, Ongoing Survival 36 Years
(Dec 1978⁻   )

Synopsis

Mr. Zhao, worker, was born in Shanghai, China. He was admitted because of elevated AFP during liver cancer survey and a space-occupying lesion in the lower part of his right liver on isotope scanning. In Dec 1978 at age 39, he was explored. The tumor 9cm located in segments V – VI of the liver with no cirrhosis and a partial hepatectomy was performed by Dr. Yeqin Yu and Dr. Xinda Zhou. Pathology report was HCC. Recovery was smooth and no adjuvant treatment administered. AFP dropped from 1,000μg/L to normal. Follow-up by Sep 2015 at age 76, he was alive and well with ongoing survival of 36 years.

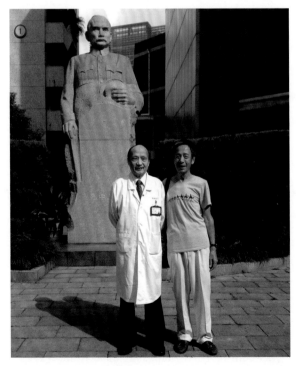

Fig. 1.19   Thirty-six years ongoing survival after a single resection. Patient (right) and his surgeon, Prof. Xinda Zhou, Sep 2015, in front of the Dr. Yatsen Sun statue at Zhongshan Hospital

Other Relevant Data

The patient's father died of liver cancer and his uncle had liver cirrhosis.

In addition to liver cancer, he also had multiple comorbidities. However, after treatment, he overcame all of them. His prostate cancer was resected at the Shanghai Tumor Hospital in 2011. He underwent radiofrequency ablation for atrial fibrillation (AF) at the Shanghai Chest Hospital in 2012. He also received a right hernia repair in 2013.

Although encountered various difficulties, he was able to deal with them properly. He loved life, enjoyed travelling and realized his wishes. He also liked to participate in social activities, share anticancer experiences and transfer positive attitudes to benefit fellow patients.

He had a wide-range of food options, with no specific food preferences or dietary restrictions.

Key Points to Remember

This case illustrated once again that long-term survival of patients depended not only on treatment of the cancer, but also on appropriate management of comorbidities. If the results of prostatectomy and radiofrequency ablation for AF were poor, he would not have survived this long.

Case 19

(Admission No. 144829)
A Single Resection, Total Survival 29 Years
(Aug 1979–Aug 2008)

Synopsis

Ms. Jiang was born in Wuxi, Jiangsu, China. In the 1970s, advanced imaging equipments were not widely available. She was admitted because of elevated AFP during liver cancer survey. Although no space-occupying lesion was found on isotope liver scanning, liver cancer was still highly suspected. In Aug 1979 at age 53, she was explored. A 6cm tumor located in the right posterior lobe of the liver and a partial hepatectomy was performed by Dr. Zhaoyou Tang and Dr Xinda Zhou. Pathology report was HCC. Recovery was smooth and no adjuvant treatment administered. AFP dropped from 1,000μg/L to normal. Unfortunately, in the 29th post-op year, Aug 2008 at age 82, she died of cerebral hemorrhage.

Other Relevant Data

Ms. Jiang had a hepatitis history but no family history of liver cancer.

In Mar 1981, after $1^1/_2$ years of liver resection, AFP rose again to 800μg/L, type-B ultrasound and hepatic angiography showed a suspicious space-occupying lesion in the liver. Strangely, no liver mass was found on laparotomy and cholecystectomy was performed for cholelithiasis. Amazingly, her AFP turned negative after surgery.

She had 3 malignancies. Except liver cancer, she also suffered from thyroid and breast cancer. In May 1968, she received a right radical mastectomy. In Jul 1968 she had a thyroidectomy. Outcome of the two procedures was satisfactory.

Key Points to Remember

This is the 3rd successful case of surgical exploration based on abnormal AFP alone. At that time, imaging studies were primitive and insensitive, operation was based only on a high index of suspicion. Today, we do not advocate any more blind abdominal exploration.

This case illustrated once again long-term survival and longevity of liver cancer patients depended not only on treatment of the liver cancer, but also on effective management of comorbidities. If outcomes of the breast and thyroid cancer were poor, the patient would not have such a long-term survival.

Through this case, we recognized that in addition to liver cancer, other diseases could also be associated with an elevated AFP. The second elevation in AFP was caused by gallstones.

Our experience is that AFP is a highly specific maker for HCC. However, other diseases, such as digestive tract tumors and cholelithiasis, etc could also cause elevation of AFP.

When AFP rises again after liver cancer resection, we should first think of recurrence or metastatic spread. When these are excluded, other diseases should be considered, although the probability is very rare. In case of doubt, the patient should be followed with imaging studies closely instead of prompt exploration.

No matter what kind of tumor we encountered, our motto is "never-say-die". Each malignancy should be taken as a separate entity de novo and managed appropriately. This case is a good illustration. She survived 29 years after liver cancer resection and 40 years after breast cancer resection.

Case 20

(Admission No. 152842)
A Single Resection, Ongoing Survival 35 Years
(Sep 1980–)

Synopsis

Mr. Sun was born in Nanjing, Jiangsu, China. He came to Zhongshan Hospital because of upper abdominal discomfort and positive AFP. Hepatic angiography showed a suspicious malignant lesion. In Sep 1980 at age 30, he was explored. The 3.5cm tumor located in the left medial lobe of the liver beside the gallbladder and a partial liver resection of the left medial lobe with cholecystectomy was performed by Dr. Zhaoyou Tang and Dr. Yeqin Yu. Pathology report was HCC. AFP dropped from 6,000μg/L to normal. In addition to oral 5-FU and FT207, Chinese Herbal Medicine was administered for 2 years. Follow-up by Sep 2015 at age 65, he led a well regulated life with ongoing survival of 35 years.

Other Relevant Data

Mr. Sun had a hepatitis history but no family history of liver cancer.

He was very optimistic and kindhearted.

He had no bad habits and no specific food preferences or dietary restrictions.

Key Points to Remember

Hepatic artery angiography is a good imaging study for locating liver cancer. Its sensitivity is higher than type-A ultrasound or isotope scanning, but the disadvantage is that it is invasive. With the advent of advanced imaging equipments, it is now infrequently used.

Case 21

(Admission No. 153219)
A Single Resection, Ongoing Survival 35 Years
(Sep 1980–   )

Synopsis

Ms. Ni was born Jan 1937, in Haimen, Jiangsu, China. In Aug 1980, she came to Zhongshan Hospital due to a palpable upper abdominal mass. AFP was positive and type-A ultrasound as well as isotope liver scanning showed a space-occupying lesion. Liver cancer was highly suspected. In Sep 1980 at age 44, she underwent exploration. Two tumors were found, one was 7.5cm located in the left lateral lobe with tumor thrombus in the left portal vein and extended into the main trunk. The other was 3cm located in the left medial lobe. A left lateral segmentectomy with removal of the tumor thrombus intact and *in toto* was performed and the tumor in the left medial lobe was laser vaporized by Dr. Yeqin Yu and Dr. Nanqiao Zhou. Pathology report was HCC. Post-op recovery was smooth and no adjuvant treatment given. AFP dropped from 80,000μg/L to normal. Follow-up by Sep 2015 at age 78, she was healthy with ongoing survival of 35 years.

Other Relevant Data

Ms. Ni was healthy before she developed liver cancer. Her family did not have any hepatic disease background.

She was cheerful and liked to share anticancer experiences with fellow patients.

In our series, the majority of patients consumed the common variety of foods, but this lady did not like chicken, duck, mutton, beef or seafood...

Her husband, two sons and grand children are healthy and happy.

Key Points to Remember

HCC is either AFP positive or AFP negative with the former being predominant. According to AFP levels, patients can arbitrarily be categorized as: ① lowly elevated AFP (>20–200μg/L); ② moderately elevated AFP (>200–10,000μg/L) ; ③ highly elevated AFP (>10,000μg/L) subgroups. Her AFP was 80,000μg/L (>10,000μg/L), evidently she belonged to the highly elevated AFP subgroup. From our experiences, there is no correlation between AFP level and prognosis.

The real value of AFP is manifested in post-op follow-up. It is used to detect recurrence, metastatic spread, monitor progression of residual disease and guide application of adjuvant therapy.

Laser vaporization is similar to resection. Microwave, radiofrequency ablation, ethanol injection, cryotherapy, etc. are all tumorcidal. However, Laser vaporization needs sophisticated advanced equipment and technology, has now been abandoned.

Cancer can invade blood vessels, forming tumor thrombus. Based on location, tumor thrombi could be in the portal vein, bile duct, hepatic vein and inferior vena cava. Presence of thrombus denotes progression of the disease, but does not necessarily contraindicate surgery. Localized thrombus and even when extended into the main trunk or an important branch can still be salvaged. When hepatic resection with removal of the tumor thrombus intact and *in toto* is performed, a curative result could be expected.

We feel that there is no scientific basis to avoid certain foods to enhance the good outcome after treatment. These is no relationship between efficacy and diet. In our series, more than 80% of patients ingested freely the common foods.

Hepatitis is contagious, but liver cancer is not. A liver cancer patient does not need to be isolated from his/her family.

Case 22

(Admission No. 151154)
Two-Step Resection and Resection of Recurrence, Ongoing
Survival 35 Years
(Jun1980-   )

Synopsis

Mr. Zhu was born Oct 1935, in Fujian, China. He came to Zhongshan Hospital due to upper abdominal discomfort. AFP was positive, type-B ultrasound, isotope liver scanning and hepatic angiography showed a space-occupying lesion denoting liver cancer. He had 3 surgeries in succession. In Jun 1980 at age 45, he underwent exploration. The 12cm huge tumor located in the middle of the right lobe with no liver cirrhosis. Diagnosis by needle biopsy was moderately differentiated HCC. After careful assessment, it was decided to perform a hepatic artery procedure instead of resection. Ligation with cannulation of the right hepatic artery was carried out by Dr Yeqin Yu and Dr. Xinda Zhou. Post-op FUDR intra-arterial chemotherapy, Cisplatin intravenous chemotherapy and oral Chinese Herbal Medicine were administered. Five months later, a miracle occurred. The tumor shrank to 6cm and AFP dropped from 1,250µg/L to 62µg/L. In Nov 1980, a right partial hepatectomy with cholecystectomy was performed by Dr. Yeqin Yu and Dr. Zhaoyou Tang. Texture of the tumor specimen was hard with massive necrosis. The procedure was basically smooth and recovery satisfactory. AFP dropped further from 62μg/L to normal. Five years later, unfortunately, type-B ultrasound showed a 3cm new solid lesion in the residual right lobe with normal AFP (10μg/L). In Jul 1986, he underwent a partial liver resection by Dr. Yeqin Yu and Dr. Zengchen Ma. In order to prevent further recurrence, silver clips were inserted into the surgical site to guide external irradiation therapy. A miracle again happened. Follow-up on Sep 2015 at age 80, there was no recurrence or metastatic spread with ongoing survival of 35 years.

Other Relevant Data

He had a hepatitis history with no family history of liver cancer.

He is very optimistic and kindhearted.

He has neither bad habits nor specific food preferences or dietary restrictions.

Surgeon's Profile

Prof. Yeqin Yu(1929—1996), male, was born in Guangdong, China, a senior hepatic oncology surgeon and former Vice Chairman of the Liver Cancer Institute. He graduated from China Medical University in 1955 and joined the Dept. of Surgery of Zhongshan Hospital.

Dr. Yu had devoted his life to research in liver cancer for nearly 30 years. He performed many very difficult liver resections and published over 40 paper, many of them were the earliest published in China, such as: *Resection of Small Liver Cancer* (1975), *Resection of Recurrent Liver Cancer* (1980), and *Hepatectomy for Cancer at the Hepatic Hilum* (1989). He was also a major participant in the National First Prize Award for "Progress in Science and Technology, P.R. China".

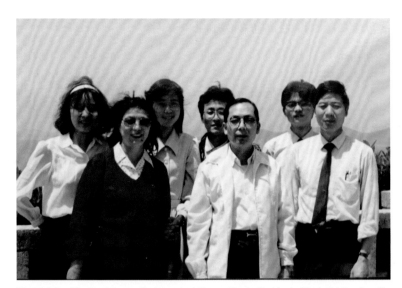

Fig. 1.20   Medical team that treated the patient. Dr. Yeqin Yu (middle, front), surgeon of the 3 successful liver operations. Photo taken in 1989

Discussion

The liver different from other organs is supplied by a dual blood supply, the hepatic artery and portal vein. Under normal conditions, blood supply comes mainly from the portal vein, but in HCC, the cancer is mainly supplied by the hepatic artery. Hepatic artery interruption provides a beneficial effect in the treatment of HCC without any adverse effect on normal activities of hepatic cells. Hepatic artery ligation (HAL) is a method of hepatic artery occlusion. Hepatic artery infusion chemotherapy (HAIC) can enhance the effect of hepatic artery ligation.

The effects of HAL and HAIC are mainly manifested in reduction of tumor volume, tumor necrosis and decreased tumor cell viability. The most ideal outcome of HAL and HAIC is to make nonresectable tumors become resectable (2-step resection), leading to long-term, high quality survival.

In some patients, a 2-step resection is better than an one-step resection, especially when the tumor is huge and surgical risks high. However, not all liver cancers are suitable for hepatic artery surgery. When requirements of a 2-step resection are fulfilled, the procedure could achieve the best result.

Key Points to Remember

He was lucky. Despite 3 surgeries, the best outcome was finally achieved. This is the most typical, most successful and longest survival case after hepatic artery surgery, a 2-step resection and resection of recurrence in this series.

As mentioned above, there is no guarantee after a 2-step resection, cancer would not recur or metastasize. Therefore, regular follow-up is still most important. In this case, if we failed to detect recurrence early and timely, the effect could not be so good.

Case 23

(Admission No. 158470)
A Single Resection, Ongoing Survival 34 Years
(Jun 1981–   )

Synopsis

Ms. Wu was born in Shandong, China. She was admitted to Zhongshan Hospital due to upper abdominal discomfort, positive AFP and a space-occupying lesion in the liver on type-B ultrasound. In Jun 1981 at age 41, she was explored. The 7cm tumor located in the right lobe and a partial liver resection was performed by Dr. Yeqin Yu and Dr. Shaoqin Zhao. Pathology report was HCC. No adjuvant treatment was administered. Recovery was uneventful and outcome satisfactory. AFP returned from 360μg/L to normal. Annual regular check-up including AFP, type-B ultrasound and chest X-ray showed no recurrence or metastasis. Follow-up by Jun 2015 at age 75, she was healthy with ongoing survival of 34 years.

Key Points to Remember

With progress of clinical research in liver cancer, many concepts have been updated. For example, the main procedure of resection is atypical resection rather than anatomic resection, especially for cancer in the right lobe. Atypical resection of the right lobe accounted for 93% in our series. The volume of liver resected is less. It not only spared more normal viable hepatic tissue, also ensured thoroughness of the resection. Ms Wu's long-term survival supported the above view.

Case 24

(Admission No. 170257)
Hepatic Artery Ligation and Cannulation with Infusion Chemotherapy, Ongoing Survival 32 Years
(Nov 1982–   )

Synopsis

Mr. Fan was born 1927, in Wuxi, Jiangsu, China. He had a 10 years hepatitis history with no family history of liver cancer. He was hospitalized due to dull upper abdominal pain, positive AFP and a space-occupying lesion in the liver on type-B ultrasound as well as isotope liver scanning. In Nov 1982 at age 55, he underwent exploration. A 10cm huge tumor located in the upper pole of the right liver close to the second hepatic hilum with moderate cirrhosis. Diagnosis by needle biopsy was HCC. After careful assessment a hepatic artery procedure was performed. Ligation with cannulation of the right hepatic artery was carried out by Dr. Yeqin Yu and Dr. Xinda Zhou. Pathology report was HCC. Three months later, hepatic artery infusion chemotherapy was discontinued due to catheter damage. Subsequently, Traditional Chinese Medicine was administered. Due to inconvenience of travel, old age and heart disease he did not return for check-up. On contact by phone, he had a wonderful outcome. AFP had dropped from 5,000µg/L to normal. Subsequent annual check-ups locally including type-B ultrasound and AFP were all normal. Follow-up by phone on May 2015 at age 88, he was alive and well with ongoing survival of 32 years.

Discussion

In general, hepatic artery ligation can lead to tumor necrosis, but does not affect viability and function of normal hepatocytes. In other words, it does not cause liver failure.

Hepatic artery procedure has many options. The site of ligation or/ and catheterization may be the hepatic artery trunk or a branch. Ligation of the main trunk would be more effective. Some scholars believe that ligation of a branch is helpful in augmenting volume of the liver remnant with reduced risk of the 2-step resection. We feel that choice of a surgical procedure should commensurate with the specific situation to bring about optimal results.

Key Points to Remember

This is the longest survival (32 years) after only hepatic artery surgery in our series. It has been proven that hepatic artery surgery is very effective in the treatment of liver cancer. In this case, we feel that hepatic artery ligation exerted a more important role in killing of the tumor, because the infusion chemotherapy duration was very short, only 3 months.

Hepatic artery ligation also has another role. In cancer with rupture and bleeding, it would control the bleeding and obviate a high risk resection or recurrent bleeding.

Case 25

(Admission No. 173983)
A Single Resection, Total Survival 30 Years
(May 1983–Jul 2013)

Synopsis

Mr. Huang, carpenter, was born in Chongming, Shanghai. He was hospitalized due to abdominal discomfort and a space-occupying lesion in the liver on type-B ultrasound and isotope liver scanning. In May 1983 at age 33, he was explored with a thoracoabdominal incision. A 16cm huge tumor located in the right lobe close to the gallbladder with moderate cirrhosis. A subtotal liver resection of the right lobe with cholecystectomy was performed by Dr. Yeqin Yu and Dr. Xinda Zhou. Pathology report was HCC. Recovery was smooth and AFP dropped from 26μg/L to normal. No adjuvant treatment was given. Unfortunately, in the 30th post-op year, in Jul 2013 at age 63, he died of liver failure due to cirrhosis.

Key Points to Remember

This case illustrated once again that long-term survival in liver cancer patients depended not only on outcome of the cancer treatment, but also on the fate of comorbidity. He would be much better off if he had no cirrhosis.

His AFP was 26μg/L, belonged to the lowly elevated AFP subgroup. According to our data, lowly elevated AFP patients are not infrequent. Usually, there is no correlation between prognosis and AFP level.

Case 26

(Admission No. 180465)
A Single Resection, Ongoing Survival 31 Years
(Feb 1984–   )

Synopsis

Mr. Chen, technician, born in Shanghai, worked in Dandong, Liaoning, China. In Sep 1983, he was explored at a local hospital, because of an acute abdomen. Operation found liver cancer rupture with bleeding. The tumor was not resected, only controlled the bleeding. Five months later, in Feb 1984 at age 52, he was admitted to Zhongshang Hospital.

The 5cm solitary tumor located in the left medial lobe close to the gallbladder without introabdominal dissemination. A partial liver resection with cholecystectomy was carried out by Dr. Yeqin Yu and Dr. Zengchen Ma. Pathology report was HCC. Recovery was smooth. Traditional Chinese Medicine was administered for 6 months. Outcome was very satisfactory. Follow-up by Sep 2015 at age 83, he was alive and healthy with ongoing survival of 31 years.

Other Relevant Data

He was healthy with no hepatitis history. His father died of variceal bleeding due to cirrhosis.

He was AFP negative and diagnosed early due to rupture of the cancer.

In addition to Traditional Chinese Medicine, no other adjuvant therapy was given.

His secret of keeping good health could be summarized as follows: correctly accepted the impact of being seriously ill, actively cooperated with the medical team and maintained an optimistic cheerful mental state.

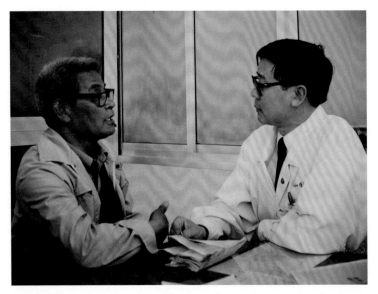 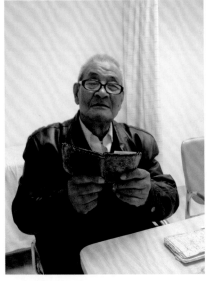

Fig. 1.21　Thirty-one years ongoing survival after liver resection. Left: Dr. Zengchen Ma and patient (May 2006, the 22nd post-op year); Right: Patient holding 30-year old outpatient medical record (Apr 2014, the 30th post-op year)

His work hours were well regulated and he liked sports, continued mountain climbing or jogging everyday.

Moreover, he paid attention to an adequate balanced diet. He has a wide choice of foods without any restrictions. In order to "improve immune function and prevent tumor recurrence", he believed in eating live insects, such as: moth, mantis, cicada, black ants, scorpion, centipede, etc.

Key Points to Remember

This case showed again that liver cancer rupture was not necessarily a bad thing and it often prompted the patient to timely seek medical care and treatment.

We do not know much of the value of eating live insects, but it is very important to ensure the food is clean and hygienic.

Case 27

(Admission No. 182114)
Two Resections, Ongoing Survival 31 Years
(Apr 1984–   )

Synopsis

Mr. Zhou, geological engineer, born in Shanghai and worked in Xian, Shaanxi, China. He was referred to Zhongshan Hospital because of whole body petechiae, thrombocytopenia, elevated AFP, type-B ultrasound and CT scan showed a space-occupying lesion in the liver. After exclusion of overt coagulopathy, in Apr 1984 at age 53, exploration revealed a 3cm tumor located in the left lateral lobe with moderate cirrhosis. A left lateral lobectomy was performed by Dr. Zhaoyu Tang and Dr. Zengchen Ma. In 1991, the 7th year after surgery, his tumor recurred. It was basically cured by 6 percutaneous ethanol injections under type-B ultrasound guidance. In 1999, AFP elevated again. B-type ultrasound and MRI showed a space-occupying lesion in the liver. In Nov 1999 at age 69, the 2.3cm recurrence located in the right lobe was resected with a right partial hepatectomy by Dr. Zengchen Ma and Dr. Qinghai Ye. The 2 pathology reports were both HCC. He continued to use interferon, Chinese Herbal Medicine, Ginseng and Ganoderma lucidum for more than 20 years. Follow-up by Sep 2015 at age 85, he was alive and well with ongoing survival of 31 years.

Other Relevant Data

He and his family had no hepatic disease background.

Pre-op AFP levels were 50μg/L and 76μg/L respectively and both dropped to normal.

He was optimistic. His work hours and family life were well regulated.

He had no bad habits or restrictions on foods.

Key Points to Remember

The pre-op AFP levels were 50μg/L and 76μg/L respectively, illustrated once again that liver cancer could have various concentrations of AFP, from less than 20μg/L to tens of thousands μg/L. It should be noted that one should not misdiagnose lowly elevated AFP as hepatitis and delay

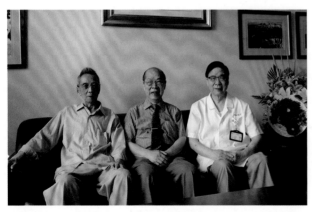

Fig. 1.22 Thirty-one years ongoing survival after two resections. Dr. Zhaoyou Tang (middle) and Dr. Zengchen Ma (right), patient (left) after the 1st operation. Sep 2015, at Zhongshan Hospital

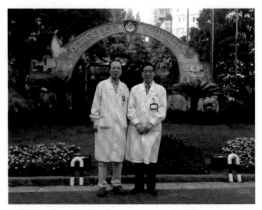

Fig. 1.23 Surgeons of the 2nd operation. Dr. Zengchen Ma (right) and Dr. Qinghai Ye in Oct 2015, at Zhongshan Hospital

treatment of liver cancer.

This is another very successful case after 2 resections. He lived another 16 years after the 2nd operation. Without which, his outcome would not necessarily be as good. Surgical resection is not the only option in treatment of recurrence, but it is the most effective.

Interferon and Traditional Chinese medicine are only adjuvant therapies.

Case 28

(Admission No. 183830)
Two Resections and Resection of Pulmonary Metastasis, Total Survival 20 Years
(Jul 1984–Apr 2004)

Synopsis

Mr. Pan, born Oct 1925, in Shicheng, Jiangxi, China. He came for check-up of discomfort in the upper abdomen. AFP was positive and type-B ultrasound as well as hepatic angiography showed a space-occupying lesion in the liver. He had 3 surgeries in succession. In Jul 1984 at age 58, the 1st exploration was by Dr. Zhaoyou Tang and Dr Zengchen Ma. A 5cm tumor located in the right posterior lobe and a partial liver resection was performed. One year later, chest X-ray revealed a 1.2cm metastatic lesion in the left upper lobe of the lung. In Aug 1985 a left upper lobectomy of the lung was performed by Dr. Zuyi Zhang and Dr. Yuanlin Shao. Six years later, a lesion in the liver was found on type-B US and CT scanning. In Oct 1991 the 3rd operation was performed by Dr. Zengchen Ma and Dr. Dongbo Xu. The 3.5cm tumor located in the left lateral lobe and a partial hepatectomy of the left lateral lobe was performed. All 3 pathology reports were HCC. Since then, no recurrence or metastasis occurred. Unfortunately, in Apr 2004 at age 78, he died of old age and frailty with 20 years survival from the first operation.

Other Relevant Data

He had a hepatitis background without family history of liver cancer.

AFP dropped from the 1st pre-op 18,000μg/L and the 2nd pre-op 200μg/L respectively to normal. However, it was negative before the 3rd operation.

Key Points to Remember

Liver cancer could have any concentration of AFP. Lowly elevated AFP (20–200μg/L) is often mistakenly ignored. With recurrence or metastasis, AFP concentration could also be different and even completely be the opposite. His 1st pre-op AFP was very high, 18,000μg/L, but less than 20μg/L before the 3rd operation. It reminds us that we should not be misled by the change in AFP concentration and forgets that AFP could change from positive to negative and vice verse with recurrence. Imaging studies should not be neglected.

This is another successful case after 3 resections. He lived 6 years after the 2nd operation and another 13 years after the 3rd. This suggested how valuable a positive attitude is in dealing with recurrence and metastasis.

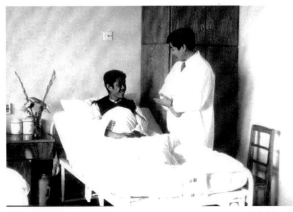

Fig. 1.24   Twenty years survival after two liver resections and resection of pulmonary metastasis. Dr. Zengchen Ma, surgeon of the liver resection and patient on 17th post-op day after the 3rd surgery in 1991

Case 29

(Admission No. 184223)
A Single Resection, Ongoing Survival 31 Years
(Jul 1984–   )

Synopsis

Mr. Tang, Traditional Chinese Medicine Practitioner, was born in Shanghai and worked in Dezhou, Shandong, China. He had hepatitis

12 years ago. There was no family history of liver cancer. He was admitted due to upper abdominal discomfort, elevated AFP and a space-occupying lesion in the liver on type-B ultrasound. In Jul 1984 at age 49, exploration revealed a 4cm tumor in the right anterior lobe beside the gallbladder. A partial liver resection with cholecystectomy was performed by Dr. Yeqin Yu and Dr Yiren Zhao. Pathology report was HCC. Recovery was smooth and outcome very satisfactory. AFP dropped from 3,000μg/L to normal. Follow-up by Sep 2015 at age 79, he was alive and well with ongoing survival of 31 years.

Key Points to Remember

This is a case with over 30 years survival. It tells us once again how crucial it is to perform early curative resection in liver cancer.

Case 30

(Admission No. 185260)
A Single Resection, Total Survival 21 Years
(Sep 1984–Oct 2005)

Synopsis

Ms. Yang was born in Shanghai and worked in Xinjiang, China. She had a hepatitis history but no family history of liver cancer. She was asymptomatic, but had elevated AFP on liver cancer survey. Type-B ultrasound and isotope liver scanning showed a space-occupying lesion in the liver. In Sep 1984 at age 62, she was operated on by Dr. Zhaoyou Tang and Dr Zengchen Ma. A 3.5cm tumor located in the upper pole of the right liver with mild cirrhosis. A partial liver resection was performed. Pathology report was HCC. Recovery was smooth and outcome satisfactory. AFP dropped from 1,040μg/L to normal. Unfortunately, In Oct 2005 at age 83, she died of renal failure though survived tumor-free for 21 years.

Key Points to Remember

As for the therapeutic effect of liver cancer, this is a very successful case. Unfortunately, due to renal failure her life did not further extend.

Case 31

(Admission No. 185172)
A Single Resection, Total Survival 26 Years
(Sep 1984–Jul 2010)

Synopsis

Mr. Xiong was born in Suqian, Jiangsu, China. He had a 23 years hepatitis history with no family history of liver cancer. He was asymptomatic, but AFP-positive during liver cancer survey. Type-B ultrasound showed a space-occupying lesion in the left lobe of the liver. Strangely, the lesion could not be detected on CT scan. In Sep 1984 at age 51, he was explored by Dr. Yeqin Yu and Dr Zengchen Ma. A 2cm tumor was in the left lateral lobe of the liver with moderate cirrhosis. A left lateral segmentectomy was performed. Pathology was HCC. Recovery was smooth and no adjuvant treatment given. AFP dropped from 1,040μg/L to normal. Unfortunately, in Jul 2010 at age 77, the 26th post-op year, he died of metastasis to the brain.

Physician's Profile

Prof. Binghui Yang was born Aug 1938 in Zhenjiang, Jiangsu, China, a senior Hepatic Oncology physician, former Director of Zhongshan Hospital and Vice Chairman of the Liver Cancer Institute. He graduated from the Shanghai First Medical College in 1962 and became a physician at his Alma Mater. He was a major participant in "Study on Small Hepatocellular Carcinoma" that won "the National First Prize Award for Progress in Science and Technology, P.R. China" (1985).

Dr. Yang has devoted his life to research in hepatocellular carcinoma

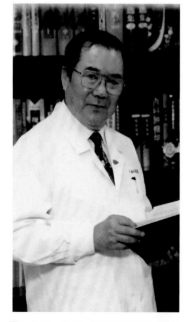

Fig. 1.25 Prof. Binghui Yang. This patient was screened and detected by Dr. Yang's medical team to have a small liver cancer and survived 26 years after resection

for more than 30 years. His main research was early detection and early diagnosis of liver cancer. He was one of the leading advocates and leaders of liver cancer screening in Shanghai and China. His medical team had detected many small liver cancers and urged the patients to undergo surgical treatment to achieve a good or the best result. Mr. Xiong was one of the small liver cancer patients screened and detected by his medical team.

He is a peaceful, simple and humble physician, as well as a health educator and pen painter.

Key Points to Remember

Type-B ultrasound and CT scan are very advanced diagnostic tools. They can detect very small even 1 cm space-occupying lesions. They often are complementary, and make up for each other's deficiency, minimizing misdiagnosis and missed diagnosis. This patient's tumor was not the smallest (2cm), but could not be found on CT scan. Fortunately, complementary type-B ultrasound imaging detected the lesion. We feel whenever liver cancer is suspected, it is best to perform both, type-B ultrasound imaging and CT scan or MRI.

Lung metastasis is not uncommon. Some are still treatable, and even be salvageable. It is important to detect early and promptly apply active treatment. Adrenal metastasis or bone metastasis is infrequent. Brain metastasis is very rare and prognosis poor. How to detect these early and start effective treatment needs further study.

Case 32

(Admission No. 187082)
Two-Step Resection, Total Survival 26 Years
(Dec1984–Sep 2011)

Synopsis

Mr. Zhang was born in Anhui, China. He had no hepatitis history or family history of liver cancer. During routine health examination, AFP was positive and type-B ultrasound found a space-occupying lesion in the liver. In Dec 1984 at age 57, exploration revealed a 2.5cm tumor in the upper pole of the right lobe, less than 1 cm from the inferior vena cava. The liver was mildly cirrhotic. Diagnosis by needle biopsy was HCC. After careful assessment, cryotherapy was performed by Dr. Zhaoyou Tang and Dr Yanming Bao. No adjuvant therapy was given. Nine months later, the tumor shrank to 1.7cm with clear boundary and AFP dropped from 5,000µg/L to 260µg/L. In Sep 1985, a right partial liver resection was performed by Dr. Zhaoyou Tang and Dr. Zengchen Ma. The resection was basically smooth and recovery satisfactory. After resection, AFP dropped to normal. Unfortunately, 25 years later, in Sep 2011 at age 84, he died of recurrence, because he neglected regular follow-ups and missed opportunities of needed further treatment.

Key Points to Remember

This is another 2-step resection case. The first step was cryotherapy and the second, liver resection.

When and how to perform a 2-step resection depends on the patient's status, tumor character, available instruments and equipments as well as the surgeon's experience and expertise.

In general, hepatic artery surgery is applicable in the 2-step resection of large HCC, small HCC with severe cirrhosis or those located in the hepatic hilum where resection has high risks. The following are alternative treatment options: hepatic artery surgery, various local treatments and TACE.

Local treatments include cryosurgery, radiofrequency ablation, ethanol injection, microwave, etc. For unknown reasons cryosurgery had been abandoned.

This patient's tumor was not big, but located close to the inferior vena cava. It was suitable for cryotherapy with less risk. After treatment, the tumor shrank away from the inferior vena cava and was safely resected. In general, HCC exceeding 5cm is not suitable for cryotherapy.

Case 33

(Admission No. 188082)
A Single Resection, Total Survival 28 Years
(Jan 1985–Nov 2013)

Synopsis

Mr. Guo, worker, was born in Jiangyin, Jiangsu and worked in Shanghai. He had a hepatitis history of 14 years but no family history of liver cancer. He was asymptomatic, but AFP positive during physical check-up. Type-B ultrasound and hepatic angiography showed a space-occupying lesion in the right liver. However, the lesion could not be detected on CT scan. In Jan 1985 at age 50, he was explored. A 1.4cm tumor located in the right lobe with moderate cirrhosis. A partial liver resection was performed by Dr. Zhaoyou Tang and Dr. Zengchen Ma. Pathology was HCC. Recovery was smooth and no adjuvant treatment given. His AFP dropped from 3,000μg/L to normal. Unfortunately, in Nov 2013 at age 79, the 28th post-op year, he died of recurrence and metastases to both lungs.

Key Points to Remember

This is another very successful case. His tumor was the smallest (1.4cm) in our series. With AFP assay, advanced imaging equipment and skillful surgical technique, the tumor was detected early, resected promptly and thoroughly. Ultimately he survived for more than 20 years.

Regrettably, he was too optimistic about his outcome and believed he was completely cured. He ignored regular check-up and lost the chance of early detection with timely treatment of recurrence and metastasis.

When AFP-positive patient has a recurrence, AFP usually becomes again elevated. However, with some recurrence AFP does not necessarily remain positive and loses its value as a monitor of the course of the disease. Hence, imaging studies become very important.

If not implemented, a normal AFP could create a false sense of security that often leads to a disastrous outcome. This patient illustrated this situation, AFP was still negative (only 14.8μg/L) when the tumor recurred.

Our experience is that tumor size has no direct relationship with the level of AFP. Both size and the latter have no correlation with prognosis.

Case 34

(Admission No. 189063)
A Single Resection, Ongoing Survival 30 Years
(Mar 1985–   )

Synopsis

Mr. He was born in Zhejiang, China. He had hepatitis 2 years ago, but no family history of liver cancer. He was admitted for upper abdominal discomfort, AFP 8,000μg/L and a space-occupying lesion in the liver on type-B ultrasound. In Mar 1985 at age 42, exploration revealed a 2.8cm tumor located in the right posterior lobe with no cirrhosis. A partial liver resection was performed by Dr. Zhaoyou Tang and Dr. Zengchen Ma. Pathology was HCC. Recovery was smooth and outcome was satisfactory. AFP dropped to normal. Follow-up by May 2015 at age 72, he was alive and well with ongoing survival of 30 years.

Key Points to Remember

This case illustrated once again there is no direct relationship between tumor size and AFP level. Small liver cancer could be accompanied by high levels of AFP and vice versa.

Case 35

(Admission No.194916)
Hepatic Artery Ligation and Cannulation with Infusion
Chemotherapy, Total Survival 25 Years
(Dec1985–Aug2010)

Synopsis

Mr. Liu was born in Hunan and worked in Shandong, China. He had a hepatitis history, but no family history of liver cancer. He was admitted for positive AFP on cancer survey and a space-occupying lesion in the liver on type-B ultrasound. In Dec 1985 at age 48, exploration revealed a 6cm tumor in the left lateral lobe with severe cirrhosis and splenomegaly. Diagnosis by needle biopsy was HCC. Normally, a left lateral lobectomy would be performed when without or only mild cirrhosis. After careful assessment, a relatively minor procedure, ligation with cannulation of the left hepatic artery and splenectomy were performed by Dr. Zhaoyou Tang and Dr. Liming Li. The procedure was basically smooth and recovery uneventful. The cancer was controlled and AFP dropped from 1,000μg/L to normal. Unfortunately, his life was curtailed by renal failure. In Aug 2010 at age 73, he died with a total survival of 25 years.

Key Points to Remember

This was the second successful case that survived for more than 20 years after simply hepatic artery surgery in our series.

Hepatic artery surgery included hepatic artery ligation and cannulation. Hepatic artery ligation is a direct blow on tumor growth. The site of ligation could be the main trunk (proper or common hepatic artery), its branch (left or right hepatic artery) or both. Although hepatic artery cannulation does not directly affect tumor growth, it provided a channel to administer chemotherapy directly to the tumor. The site of catheterization should be at the proper hepatic artery (not common hepatic artery) or its branch (left or right hepatic artery). In this patient, ligation with catheterization was the left hepatic artery as the tumor located on the left side and outcome of the ligation equated that of radical resection.

It was also most regrettable, kidney failure ended his life.

Case 36

(Admission No. 195978)
A Single Resection, Ongoing Survival 29 Years
(Jan 1986–   )

Synopsis

Ms. Sun was born in Shanghai, China. She and her family had no hepatic disease background. In Jan 1983, she underwent bilateral ovariectomy and salpingo-hysterectomy for teratoma of the ovary. Recovery was smooth and outcome satisfactory. Three years later, check-up found a positive AFP and space-occupying lesion in the liver on type-B ultrasound and isotope scanning. In Jan 1986 at age 27, exploration revealed a 3.1cm tumor located in the left lateral lobe with no cirrhosis. A left lateral lobectomy was performed by Dr. Yeqin Yu and Dr. Baoquan Jia. Pathology was HCC. Outcome was very satisfactory. AFP dropped from 450μg/L to normal. Follow-up by May 2015 at age 56, she was alive and well for 29 years with no recurrence or metastasis.

Key Points to Remember

She had two different tumors in succession and underwent 2 major operations.

She was fortunate as her physicians paid attention to regular follow-ups and monitored tumor markers including AFP, leading to early detection and prompt resection of liver cancer.

We should never forget that despite she lived tumor-free for 29 years, follow–up of liver cancer should not be neglected. We insist on lifelong follow-up to achieve the best outcome.

Case 37

(Admission No. 197067)
A Single Resection, Total Survival 20 Years
(Mar 1986–Dec 2005)

Synopsis

Mr. Yu was born in Zhenhai and worked in Shanghai. He and his family had no hepatic disease background. In Feb 1986, during annual check-up, type-B ultrasound and ^{99m}Tc-PMT isotope liver scanning detected a space-occupying lesion, but AFP was negative. Type-B ultrasound revealed a typical liver cancer image, exploration was suggested but refused. As he was asymptomatic nor AFP positive, after repeated exchanges and psychological counseling, he finally consented to have surgery. On Mar 28 1986 at age 49, exploration found a tumor 3.5cm in the right lobe close to the gallbladder with moderate cirrhosis. A partial liver resection with cholecystectomy was performed by Dr. Zhaoyou Tang and Zengchen Ma. Pathology was highly differentiated HCC. Recovery and outcome were satisfactory.

Twelve years later (1998), Type B ultrasound detected a very small recurrence (only 1cm) in the right liver. CT and MRI scanning further confirmed the ultrasound finding. In Oct 1999, when prepared for surgical treatment he was involved in a traffic accident. He had multiple fractures, 9 ribs, a scapula and a left tibia and fibula open fracture. He was admitted to a local tertiary trauma center and underwent 15 debridements. The recurrence, by then had increased to 11cm. In Apr 2005, at the second exploration, the tumor was located in the right posterior lobe close to the inferior vena cava with dense adhesions. Resection was abandoned. In Dec 2005, he died at age 68 with a total survival of 20 years.

Discussion

Type-B ultrasound is a very useful imaging instrument. It is able to find even an 1cm intrahepatic space-occupying lesion. It has also a strong function in differential diagnosis. It can distinguish cystic from parenchymal lesions and benign from malignant tumors. Type-B ultrasound often reveals a hypoechoic light mass with rich arterial blood flow in small liver cancer. Cirrhosis also has its own characteristic manifestations on type-B ultrasound. In view of these, even when AFP is negative, diagnosis of liver cancer is still credible.

Isotope liver scanning can be divided into two types: positive and negative. Negative liver scan shows only a focal defect. It does not show the function and nature of the space occupying lesion. On the contrary, sensitivity of a positive liver scan is high, and nature of the space occupying lesion could also be ascertained. HCC cells have the function of uptaking PMT. PMT (pyridoxy-l-5-methyl-tryptophane) is excreted by the biliary tract. ^{99m}Tc-PMT imaging could not only be used in diagnosis of biliary tract diseases, but also for HCC, especially, in highly differentiated small HCC. ^{99m}Tc-PMT imaging in this patient was positive, further supported the diagnosis of HCC.

Key Points to Remember

There are two kinds of liver cancer, primary and secondary. Pathologically, according to its cell origin, primary liver cancer can be divided into three kinds, hepatocellular carcinoma (HCC), intrahepatic cholangiocellular carcinoma and mixed hepato-cholangiocellular carcinoma. HCC can also be divided into AFP positive and negative. Usually, HCC is often rich in arterial blood supply. When type-B ultrasound, contrast enhanced ultrasound, contrast CT, contrast MRI and hepatic arteriography showed an abundant arterial blood supply in a hepatic lesion, diagnosis of HCC, should be considered.

In addition, PMT scanning is especially helpful in the diagnosis of

AFP-negative HCC.

In general, lesions other than HCC are rarely associated with cirrhosis. The presence of cirrhosis with a space-occupying lesion often suggests HCC and no other disease.

In an AFP negative patient, 3 points support a HCC diagnosis: ① cirrhosis on imaging studies, ② rich arterial blood supply and ③ positive PMT isotope scan.

This was another very lucky case. Although he had no symptoms with AFP negative, type-B ultrasound and ^{99m}Tc-PMT imaging made the diagnosis. With repeated exchanges and psychological counseling, he finally consented to have surgery and ultimately won 20 years of long-term survival.

Because of the serious traffic accident, he was treated at another hospital. The cancer problem did not alert enough attention to take priority in management.

When multiple morbidities exist, there is a need to arrange their management in sequence. The consensus is the most serious or potentially most lethal has the top priority. In other words, life saving is the supreme goal. In this case, an error in judgement allowed osteomyelitis to displace cancer from its top place. The delay in cancer treatment inevitably reaped a sad outcome.

Case 38

(Admission No. 199474)
Two-Step Resection, Ongoing Survival 29 Years
(Jun1986-   )

Synopsis

Mr. Wang, electrician, was born in May 1954, in Yangzhou, Jiangsu and worked in Shanghai. He and his family had no hepatic disease background. He came to Zhongshan Hospital due to positive AFP and a space-occupying lesion in the liver on type-B ultrasound during physical check-up. In Jun 1986 at age 32，he underwent exploration. An isolated huge 9cm tumor was located in the right lobe with mild cirrhosis. Diagnosis by needle biopsy was HCC. After careful assessment, a hepatic artery procedure, ligation with cannulation of the right hepatic artery was carried out by Dr. Zhaoyou Tang and Dr. Zengchen Ma. In addition, silver clip markers were inserted into the surgical area to guide external radiotherapy. Brachy-radiotherapy with ^{131}I-labeled anti-HCC isoferritin antibody beads as well as ^{131}I-labeled anti-HCC monoclonal antibody beads via the right hepatic artery were given. Five months later, a miracle occurred. The tumor shrank to 4cm and AFP dropped from 690μg/L to 100μg/L. In Nov 1986, the 2nd operation, a partial liver resection was performed by Dr. Zengchen Ma. Texture of the tumor specimen was hard and 85% was necrotic. The procedure was basically smooth and recovery satisfactory. AFP dropped to normal. Follow-up by Sep 2015 at age 61, the patient was alive with ongoing survival of 29 years.

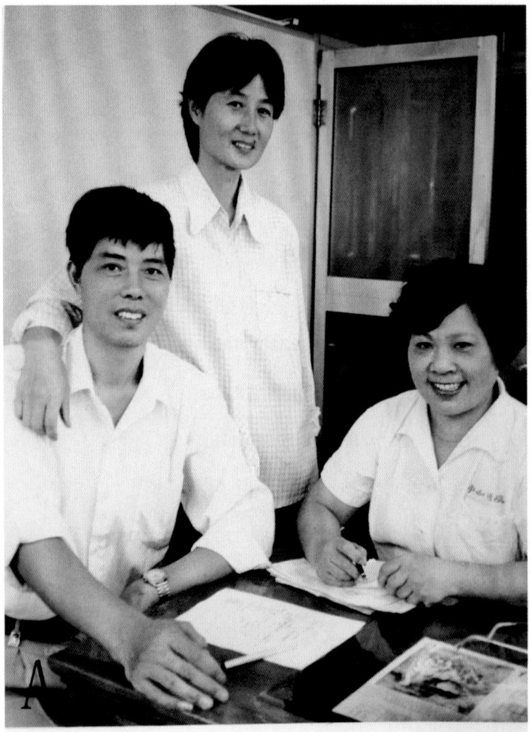

Key Points to Remember

This was the 2nd most typical, successful and longest survived case after hepatic artery surgery and a 2-step resection in our series.

This case also showed that multimodal therapy could be more effective. We feel that external irradiation therapy is only suitable for single or a relatively localized lesion, but not when multiple or diffuse. At times, it is not only useless but harmful.

There is no guarantee that there would be no recurrence or metastasis. Regular follow-up is still most important.

Fig. 1.26 Twenty-nine years ongoing survival after two-step resection. Patient (left), his wife (middle) and Ms. Lijin Lu (right), staff of Follow-up Unit of the Liver Cancer Institute, Zhongshan Hospital (1998, the 12th post-op year)

Case 39

(Admission No. 199641)
A Single Resection, Ongoing Survival 29 Years
(Aug 1986‒   )

Synopsis

Mr. Wang, teacher, was born in Jan 1941 in Taizhou, Jiangsu, China. He was healthy before he had liver cancer. He and his family did not have any hepatic disease background.

In Jun 1986 at age 45, because of discomfort around the liver area for 3 months, elevated AFP and an intrahepatic space-occupying lesion on type-B ultrasound and isotope scanning, he underwent exploration. The 9cm tumor was located in the right posterior lobe of the liver with no cirrhosis. An extended right posterior lobectomy was carried out (thoracoabdominal incision) by Dr. Zhaoyou Tang and Dr. Peile Huang. Pathology was moderately differentiated HCC. AFP dropped from 12,000μg/L to normal.

Follow-up by Sep 2015 at age 74, He was healthy with an ongoing tumor-free survival of 29 years.

Other Relevant Data

He is optimistic and lived a regulated life, paying attention to work and rest.

He has a wide-range of food options, including chicken, beef, mutton and sea food, but does not like spicy foods.

Key Points to Remember

According to tumor size, liver cancer was arbitrarily divided into small liver cancer (<5cm) and large liver cancer (>5cm). If the maximum diameter is more than 10cm, it is called a huge liver cancer, more than 15cm, a giant liver cancer. Normally, the majority of small liver cancers are early liver cancers. Small liver cancer is characterized by a relatively high resection rate and good therapeutic outcome. With increase in tumor volume, resection rate is relatively low and the curative effect relatively poor. If the large, even huge or giant liver cancer is solitary, its boundary clear, without disseminated nodules, complicating tumor thrombus and other contraindications, resection is still the first option. This patient's tumor was a 9cm large liver cancer. However, his tumor condition was not complicated and good results achieved after thorough resection.

We emphasize again, no matter how successful surgery is with a good effect, we must not neglect regular check-up to ensure the best result.

Case 40

(Admission No. 199855)
A Single Resection, Ongoing Survival 29 Years
(Jul 1986-   )

Synopsis

Mr. Qi was born in Shandong, China. He and family had no hepatic disease background. He was asymptomatic. In Jul 1986 at age 35, because of elevated AFP and an intrahepatic space-occupying lesion on type-B ultrasound, isotope and CT liver scanning during a check-up, he underwent exploration. The 3.5cm tumor located in the left medial lobe of the liver near the gallbladder with moderate cirrhosis. A left partial hepatectomy with cholecystectomy was carried out by Dr. Zhaoyou Tang and Dr. Zengchen Ma. Pathology was HCC. Recovery was smooth and outcome satisfactory. AFP dropped from 266µg/L to normal.

Follow-up for 29 years, by Sep 2015 at age 63, he was healthy and happy.

Case 41

(Admission No. 200764)
Two Resections, Ongoing Survival 29 Years
(Jul 1986–   )

Synopsis

Mr. Xing, teacher, was born Dec 1933 in Suozhou, Anhui and worked in Hangzhou, Zhejiang. He was transferred from a local hospital to Zhongshan Hospital due to positive AFP and a space-occupying lesion in the liver on type-B ultrasound during a check-up. A CT scan confirmed existence of the lesion, denoting liver cancer. In Jul 1986 at age 52, he underwent exploration. The 3cm tumor located in the right lower-posterior lobe with mild cirrhosis. A right partial liver resection was performed by Dr. Yeqin Yu and Dr. Zengchen Ma. 5-fluorouracil systemic chemotherapy and interferon were administered for less than one month. Thirteen years later, AFP was again elevated. Type-B ultrasound and CT scan found a new lesion in the liver. In Aug 1999 at age 65, he was operated on again. The 7cm tumor located in the right upper lobe of the liver, 1.5cm from the inferior vena cava. A right partial hepatectomy was performed by Dr. Zengchen Ma and Dr. Qinghai Ye. The 2 pathology diagnoses were HCC. In order to prevent further recurrence, prophylactic hepatic artery interventional treatment was administered. Follow-up by Sep 2015 at age 81, he was alive and well with ongoing survival of 29 years from the first surgery.

Other Relevant Data

He had hepatitis 7 years ago, but his family had no hepatic disease background.

He was AFP positive which dropped from 800 and 84μg/L respectively to normal after surgery.

He was a very kind and optimistic person. He liked to share with other fellow patients anticancer experiences. He was also a very serious and well respected teacher.

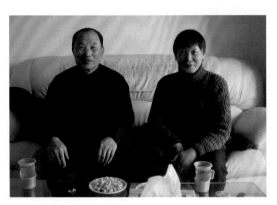

Fig. 1.27　Patient (left) and wife, 29 years ongoing survival after 2 liver resections （Dec 2007 at Shanghai）

He had no bad eating habits or restrictions on foods.

Key Points to Remember

Liver cancer is an aggressive malignancy with metastatic tendencies.

No matter how early and how small the tumor is, as well as how thorough the resection, it could not be absolutely guaranteed from recurrence or metastasis.

Regular follow-up, early detection and timely treatment of new lesions is very important in improving outcome.

This was the 4th long-term survivor after 2 hepatic resections in our series. After the 2nd resection, he survived for another 16 years or a total ongoing survival of 29 years.

Case 42

(Admission No. 202544)
Two-Step Resection and Resection of Pulmonary Metastasis, Ongoing Survival 28 Years
(Oct 1986-　)

Synopsis

Ms. Zheng was born Jul 1942, in Haimen, Jiangsu and worked in Shanghai. She was asymptomatic, but AFP elevated during a check-up and persisted for 14 months. Recent imaging on type-B ultrasound, isotope and CT liver scan showed a space-occupying lesion denoting liver cancer. She was referred to Zhongshan Hospital and had 3 surgeries in succession. The first was in Oct 1986 at age 44. Two big isolated tumors 9cm and 6cm, separately located in the right lobe (segments V – VI) and left medial lobe (segment IV) with no cirrhosis. Diagnosis by needle biopsy was HCC. After full onsite assessment, a hepatic artery procedure, ligation with cannulation of the left hepatic artery and ligation of the right hepatic artery were carried out by Dr. Zengchen Ma and Dr. Teer Ba. Subsequently, FUDR, VCR, DDP infusion chemotherapy via the left hepatic artery as well as oral Chinese Herbal Medicine were given for about 1 year. In Nov 1987, the catheter was blocked after intrahepatic embolization with Lipiodol. Thereafter, short term interferon injections and systemic chemotherapy were administered. Surprisingly, imaging found both tumors reduced to 1/3 of their original size. AFP also dropped from 580μg/L to 40μg/L. In Feb 1988, the 2nd operation was performed by Dr. Zhaoyou Tang and Dr. Zengchen Ma. Both tumors had become white scar-like tissues and shrank to 3cm and 2cm respectively, but were extremely close to the first hepatic hilum. After careful assessment liver resection was performed. The gallbladder was first removed. Then the hepatic hilum especially right hepatic duct was carefully isolated and protected. The 2 "scar-like tumors" were completely resected. The patient recovered well with no complications. AFP dropped to normal. Pathology was fibrous connective tissue with tumor necrosis.

Six years later, AFP was again elevated. Metastasis to the lung and mediastinum was confirmed. Neither of the 2 metastatic lesions was large. In Oct 1994, the 3rd operation was performed by Dr. Yunzhong

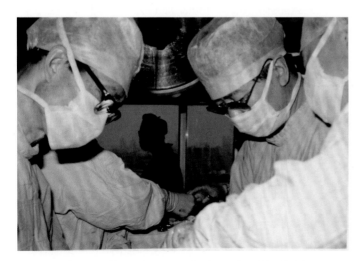

Fig. 1.28   Dr. Zhaoyou Tang（left）and Dr. Zengchen Ma (right) at operation

Zhou of the Shanghai Chest Hospital. A lesion, 0.8cm size was in the right lung, the other egg sized in the mediastinum. Right upper pulmonary lobectomy and mediastinal metastasis resection were carried out. Pathology was metastatic HCC. The patient recovered well and post-op external radiotherapy was added for 50 days. In addition, Traditional Chinese Medicine was also given for 5 years by Dr. Chenlong Tang. After the 3rd surgery she remained stable for 20 years.

In Mar 2014, ultrasound found two recurrent lesions, one 2.8cm in the right anterior lobe and another 1.4cm in the left medial lobe of the liver. These were confirmed on MRI with elevated AFP (100μg/L). In Jun 2014, radiofrequency ablation was applied to the two lesions by Dr. Ningling Ge. The procedure was successful and outcome satisfactory. Ultrasound and MRI found no blood supply to the two lesions, indicated tumor necrosis. AFP reduced to normal again. TCM, containing mainly Cinobufotalin (orally 6 ampules bid) was again given.

Follow-up by Sep 2015 at age 75, she remained stable and AFP normal with ongoing survival of 28 years.

Other Relevant Data

She had no hepatic disease history, but had a family history of liver cancer. Two of her uncles, a young brother and a young sister all died of liver cancer. Another young brother and sister are alive after resection of liver cancer or transplantation.

She had a positive attitude of life and believed in modern science. She had a warm family and all members were willing to share difficulties.

She had no bad habits and no specific food preferences or dietary restrictions.

Key Points to Remember

This was a typical AFP-positive liver cancer. All her AFP assays were positive before surgery and radiofrequency ablation. After treatment all returned

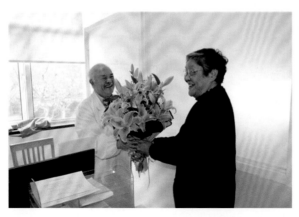

Fig. 1.29 Patient visiting Dr. Yunzhong Zhou (left) who performed the pneumonectomy and mediastinal resection (Apr 2015 at the Shanghai Chest Hospital)

to normal.

It is well known that liver cancer can be AFP-positive or AFP-negative. It should be remembered that in AFP-positive liver cancer, it is not always positive when tumor recurs. In other words, AFP-positive HCC might become AFP-negative.

This is another typical and successful case after hepatic artery surgery and 2-step resection.

We would like to emphasize that hepatic artery surgery does not necessarily always could lead to a two-step liver resection. A two-step resection of liver cancer is not a "once and for all" procedure. The best results could only be obtained by close follow-up and aggressive follow-up treatment.

Her treatments included ligation and cannulation of the hepatic artery (1986, age 44), hepatectomy (1988), pneumonectomy with mediastinal resection for metastasis (1994) and radiofrequency ablation for recurrence (2014). In addition, TCM and radiotherapy were also given. Follow-up by 2015 at age 73, she was alive and well.

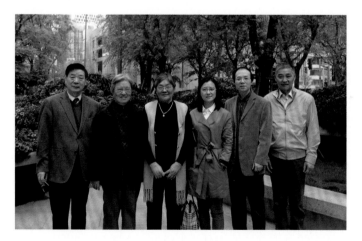

Fig. 1.30   Patient (3rd, left), long-term survivor after liver resection and her physicians: Dr. Zengchen Ma (1st, left), surgeon; Dr. Chenlong Tang (2nd, left), physician of Integrated Chinese and Western Medicine; Dr. Qinghai Ye (2nd, right), surgeon; Dr. Ningling Ge (3rd, right), physician, who performed the radiofrequency ablation; Patient's young brother (1st, right) (2015, Shanghai)

Case 43

(Admission No. 202238)
Two-Step Resection, Ongoing Survival 28 Years
(Oct 1986‒   )

Synopsis

Mr Xi, technician, born Jul 1937 in Wuxi, Jiangsu and worked in Shanghai. In Oct 1986 at age 49, he came to Zhongshan Hospital and was operated on by Dr. Zhaoyou Tang and Dr. Peile Huang for upper abdominal discomfort, positive AFP and a solid space-occupying lesion on type-B ultrasound. A 10cm×8cm×6cm huge tumor was located in the right lobe of the liver with unclear margin. Diagnosis by needle biopsy was HCC. As forceful resection would carry great risks, it was decided to ligate and cannulate the right hepatic artery. In addition, silver clips were inserted to the surgical site to guide post-op external radiotherapy. The tumor shrank to 9cm×5cm×5cm with clear margins and AFP decreased from 700µg/L to 268µg/L after intra-arterial chemotherapy and brachy-radiotherapy with ^{131}I-labeled anti-HCC isoferritin antibody beads as well as external radiotherapy. A 2-step resection, right partial hepatectomy with cholecystectomy was performed by Dr. Zhaoyou Tang and Dr. Zengchen Ma in May 1987. Pathology was fibrous connective tissue with tumor necrosis. The patient recovered well. Follow-up by Sep 2015 at age 78, he was alive and well with ongoing survival of 28 years.

Key Points to Remember

The two-step resection in liver cancer after a hepatic artery procedure needs to meet certain requirements. In principle, the tumor should have shrunken to a certain degree, to make the resection with less risk. Of course, other conditions should also be met, such as: normal liver function, good liver texture with no ascites, no new lesions, no cancer thrombosis nor distant metastasis. Efficacy of a hepatic artery procedure depends mainly on the following: degree of tumor shrinkage and necrosis, as well as compensatory hypertrophy of the residual normal liver. Usually, interval between the 2 surgeries is 3 months to a year and a half. Time is needed to maximize effect of the hepatic artery procedure.

The patient completely complied with the above conditions. Hence, the 2-step resection yielded an ideal effect.

Case 44

(Admission No. 205925)
Two Resections, Total Survival 25 Years
(Feb 1987–Dec 2012)

Synopsis

Mr. Shi was born Feb 1958 in Cangzhou, Jiangsu. The patient had hepatitis and a family history of liver cancer. His father died of liver cancer. He was referred to Zhongshan Hospital for right upper abdominal pain, elevated AFP and a solid space-occupying lesion on type-B ultrasound. He had 2 surgeries. The first was in Feb 1987 at age 29. A tumor 6.5cm×5cm×5cm was located in the middle lobe (segments VI – V) adjacent to the gallbladder and partial middle hepatectomy with cholecystectomy was performed by Dr Zhaoyou Tang and Dr. Zengchen Ma. Pathology was HCC. The tumor recurred after 10 months and was operated in Dec 1987. Two isolated tumors, 4.5cm and 1.5cm, separately located in the caudate lobe and left lateral lobe. Resection of the caudate and left lateral lobes was performed by Dr. Zengchen Ma and Dr. Lianru Zhang. Pathology again confirmed HCC. The patient remained well for 23 years. He was busy with business and ignored follow-up. A huge liver tumor with thrombi in the portal vein was detected in 2011. He lost the chance for further treatment and died of recurrence in Dec 2012 at age 54 with survival of 25 years.

Key Points to Remember

This was another very regrettable case. Result of the surgery was very good, but neglect of regular follow-up led to serious consequences and failed to further prolong his life.

Case 45

(Admission No. 264861)
Two Resections, Ongoing Survival 28 Years
(Mar 1987–   )

Synopsis

Mr. Xu was born Feb 1956 in Shanghai. He had HBV infection, but no family history of liver cancer. He was asymptomatic. In Mar 1987 at age 31 he was operated on for gallstones by Dr. Quanxing Ni of the Shanghai Huashan Hospital. During cholecystectomy, liver cancer was found incidentally. The 2cm tumor located in the right lower corner of the liver and a right partial hepatectomy was also performed. Pathology was HCC. He remained well for 6 years. In 1993, follow-up AFP was elevated (204μg/L). A solid space-occupying lesion showed on CT scanning, but repeated B-ultrasound did not reveal any lesion. In Jun 1993 at age 37 the 2ⁿᵈ surgery was performed at Zhongshan Hospital. The tumor was buried 2cm deep in the liver and its texture was similar to that of the parenchyma. Resection met with difficulty. Location of the lesion was ascertained by reading the CT scan and tactile sensing. A right partial hepatectomy was carried out by Dr. Zengchen Ma and Dr. Xiaomin Wang. The tumor was actually 2.3cm. AFP decreased to normal. Pathology report was HCC. A two-month course of interferon injection and one-year TCM were given. He recovered well and was back to work after 3 months. Regular follow-ups with AFP, B-US and chest X-ray did not detect any recurrence or metastasis. By Sep 2015 at

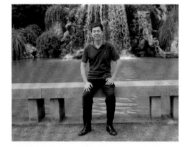

Fig. 1.31 Patient, 28 years ongoing survival after 2 resections (Sep 2014 at Xi Jiao Guest House, Shanghai)

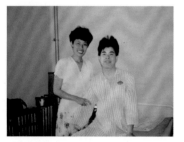

Fig. 1.32 Patient (right) and wife on the 12ᵗʰ post-op day after the 2ⁿᵈ resection (Jun 1993, age 37)

age 59, he survived 28 years and was still well and at work.

Towards Happiness

Great progress has been made in the treatment of liver cancer in China, from incurable to become curable and from short-term survival to long-term survival. Our goal is to make liver cancer patients lead a good quality normal life, just like any healthy person. Although this patient suffered great mental stress and the pains of two surgeries, he finally won the battle against cancer and enjoyed the pleasure of work and the joys of home life. At present, he is in good health and has a well-paid job. His wife though retired, is in good health and has a rich and colorful life. His son went to college and abroad for further studies and is now an airline pilot (his son was 2 years old when he had his first operation). His son is now married and has a lovely baby. The three generations are well and live happily.

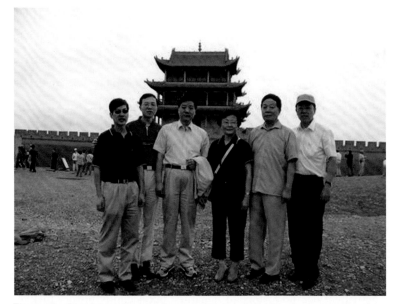

Fig. 1.33   Physicians that took care of the patient. Dr. Zengchen Ma, liver surgeon (3rd, left); Dr. Quanxing Ni, general surgeon (2nd, right) of Huashan Hospital; Dr. Zhiying Lin, internist (3rd, right); Dr. Jinglin Xia, internist (1st,left); Dr. Qinghai Ye, liver surgeon (2nd,left); Dr. Yong Zhang, general surgeon (1st,right) (Aug 2004, at Jiayuguan, Gansu,China)

Case 46

(Admission No. 206892)
Two Resections, Total Survival 27 Years
(Mar 1987–Feb 2014)

Synopsis

Mr. Wu was born Mar 1942 in Wujin, Jiangsu, China. He was asymptomatic, but AFP positive (516μg/L) with a space-occupying lesion in the liver on type-B ultrasound and CT scan during check-up. He was referred to Zhongshan Hospital and received his first surgical treatment in Mar 1987 at age 45. The 4.5cm tumor located in the left lateral lobe (segments II – III) with moderate cirrhosis and a left lateral lobectomy was smoothly performed by Dr. Zhaoyou Tang and Dr. Zengchen Ma. Pathology was moderately differentiated HCC with nodular cirrhosis. Thirteen years later, a new lesion with imaging features of liver cancer was discovered on type-B ultrasound and confirmed by CT scan, but AFP was normal (only 2μg/L). In Jan 2000 at age 58, the 2nd operation was performed. The tumor 4.5cm located in the right lobe and a right partial hepatectomy was carried out by Dr. Zengchen Ma and Dr. Qinghai Ye. Pathology was grade- II differentiated HCC. After the 2nd operation, Chinese Herbal Medicine and interferon injections were given. In Aug 2010, he had a splenectomy for splenomegaly. Unfortunately, at the end of 2013, his cancer again recurred and with ascites, pancytopenia (HGB, 63g/L; WBC, $2.5×10^9$/L; PLT, $68×10^9$/L). In Feb 2014 at age 72, he died of multiple organ failure and tumor recurrence with a total survival of 27 years.

Other Relevant Data

The patient had no history of hepatitis, but a family history of liver cancer. His father died of liver cancer in 1986.

He was AFP-positive (516μg/L) prior to the 1st operation and dropped to normal after resection. But with confirmed recurrence, AFP was only 2μg/L.

In his troubled life, he received 5 operations:

- Hepatectomy for liver cancer in 1987.
- Appendectomy for appendicitis in 1990.
- Hepatectomy for recurrence in 2000.
- Cholecystectomy in 2003.
- Splenectomy for splenomegaly in 2010.

Key Points to Remember

(1) The patient is both lucky and unfortunate. He survived 27 years after surgeries for liver cancer and repeated cancer recurrence, but because of liver failure, we failed to prolong his life.

(2) The biologic characteristics of liver cancer is not set in stone. AFP-positive HCC might become AFP-negative during recurrence and rice versa. Acknowledgement of this characteristic is helpful for early detection of tumor recurrence. His condition was in accordance with this change. He was AFP-positive, but became AFP-negative on recurrence. Recurrence would have been overlooked without ultrasound examination. Recurrence was detected early and removed in time in 2000.

(3) To date, there is no effective treatment for severe cirrhosis, except liver transplantation.

Case 47

(Admission No. 209461)
Liver Resection and Hepatic Vein Cancer Thrombectomy,
Ongoing Survival 28 Years
(Jun 1987–   )

Synopsis

Mr. Zheng, lawyer, was born Jun 1930 in Shandong, worked in

Heilongjiang. He was referred to Zhongshan Hospital due to right upper abdominal discomfort and a solid space-occupying lesion in the liver on type-B ultrasound. Diagnosis of liver cancer was based on ultrasound and ^{99m}Tc-PMT isotope liver scanning. In Jun 1987 at age 57, exploration revealed a 12cm huge liver cancer in the left lateral lobe with thrombus in the left hepatic vein. As he had enough residual liver with no severe cirrhosis, an En Bloc left hemihepatectomy including removal of the cancer thrombus was performed by Dr. Yeqin Yu and Dr. Zengchen Ma. The procedure was complicated, but resection was thorough and could be considered radical. Pathology was HCC. Interferon injections were given for 1 month. His wound infection healed uneventfully. He recovered well and went to work 6 months later. Follow-up by Sep 2015 at age 85, he was healthy with ongoing survival of 28 years. Although he was 85 years old, he had a clear mind, a loud voice and often used to take walking as exercise.

Other Relevant Data

He had no history of hepatitis or family history of liver cancer.

This was an AFP-negative case. Diagnosis was by ultrasound and ^{99m}Tc-PMT isotope liver scanning.

He was optimistic, believed in modern science and actively cooperated with his physicians. He was willing to share his experiences with other patients.

He had given up smoking and drinking and turned to soybean milk since operation.

He appreciated the concept of keeping fit: happy mood, proper nutrition, medication supplement and appropriate exercise. He did not like taking too many drugs and felt too much medication would aggravate the burden on his liver.

He had no bad habits, no specific food preferences and no dietary restrictions.

He has 7 children and his family is thriving with four generations. By May 2015 at age 85, he was still healthy leading a happy and joyful life.

Key Points to Remember

This is the 2nd long-term survivor after En-Bloc huge liver cancer resection, including removal of cancer thrombus in the left hepatic vein in our series.

We feel it is worthwhile for some liver cancer cases with cancer thrombus to carry out En Bloc radical resection including the thrombus. Such cases should be in accordance with the following conditions: good liver texture, clear tumor boundary and thrombus that can be easily removed intact and *in toto*.

Patient underwent En-Bloc left hemihepatectomy with removal of cancer thrombus in the left hepatic vein Jun 1987 at age 57.

Follow-up by Sep 2015 at age 85, he was living and well with ongoing survival for 28 years.

Case 48

(Admission No. 209800)
Liver Resection and Bile Duct Cancer Thrombectomy, Total Survival 25 Years
(Jul 1987–Dec 2012)

Synopsis

Ms. Li, was born in Panjin, Liaoning. She had no history of viral hepatitis or family history of liver cancer. She came to Zhongshan Hospital for right upper abdominal discomfort, positive-AFP (432μg/L) and a space-occupying lesion in the liver on type-B ultrasound. Her surgery was in Jul 1987 at age 32. The 3cm tumor located in the left medial lobe of the liver (segment VI) with cancer thrombus in the left bile duct and the common bile duct. As the tumor was not large and the cancer thrombus not complicated, an En Bloc left hemihepatectomy with removal of the cancer thrombus and choledochostomy with T-tube drainage were performed by Dr. Yeqin Yu and Dr. Chuanyuan Du. Pathology was HCC. Recovery was satisfactory and AFP dropped to normal. Unfortunately, she died of recurrence in Dec 2012 at age 57 due to financial difficulties and non-adherence of regular follow-up.

Key Points to Remember

Liver cancer with portal vein thrombus is quite common, but bile duct thrombus is rare. The suitability of resection in HCC patients with cancer thrombus cannot be generalized. It is not absolutely contraindicated. Surgical treatment can be considered when the thrombus is not complex and can be completely removed. In this patient, if untreated by surgery, prognosis could not be as good.

Usually, 95%–98% of liver cancer are HCC. There is no relation between hepatocellular liver cancer and cholangiocellular liver cancer. Cholangiocarcinoma is not generally associated with tumor thrombus in the bile duct. In other words, liver cancer with bile duct thrombus is not a characteristic feature of cholangiocellular liver cancer, but that of HCC.

Case 49

(Admission No. 210251)
A Single Resection, Ongoing Survival 28 Years
(Aug 1987–   )

Synopsis

Ms Fan was born Dec 1946, in Shanghai and worked in Anhui. She had no history of hepatitis, but a family history of liver cancer. Her mother and elder brother both died of liver cancer. She was referred to Zhongshan Hospital due to right upper abdomen discomfort, positive AFP (627µg/L) and a space-occupying lesion on type-B ultrasound. In Aug 1987 at age 40, she was explored. A tumor 4cm in the right lobe of the liver close to the right bile duct, classified as hilar liver cancer was found. A right partial liver resection was performed by Dr. Yeqin Yu and

Dr. Fahong Zheng. After removal of the tumor, a small bile leak on the liver cut surface was sutured. Pathology was HCC. In order to facilitate healing of the bile duct leak, a T-tube was placed in the common bile duct. AFP dropped to normal. Two months later the bile leak healed and T-tube removed. Since then, her recovery was smooth and outcome satisfactory. By Sep 2015, she was 68 years old and still healthy with ongoing survival of 28 years.

Key Points to Remember

Ms. Fan is one of those who agree with the view that chicken could induce tumor recurrence. She never ate chicken after the operation. We feel that liver cancer patients need nutrition to protect the liver and improve immunity, 70%–90% of our long-term survivals are not prohibited to eat chicken, mutton and seafood. The above view "some foods could induce tumor recurrence" is unscientific.

Bile leak is one of the complications after liver resection. Resection of cancer near the first hepatic hilum is more likely to be associated with bile leak. It is possible to reduce the incidence of bile leak by careful dissection and protection of the large bile duct with firm ligation or suturing of the small bile duct. If injury of the bile duct is unavoidable, a good way to reduce postoperative complications is by placing a T-tube in the common bile duct at operation.

Case 50

(Admission No. 210022)
Liver Resection and Portal Vein Cancer Thrombectomy,
Ongoing Survival 27 Years
(Sep 1987–　)

Synopsis

Mr. Li was born in Jiangsu. He had no history of hepatitis or family history of liver cancer. He was referred to Zhongshan Hospital for right upper abdominal pain and elevated AFP (500μg/L). All imaging studies, including type-B ultrasound, ^{99m}Tc-PMT isotope and CT liver scan failed to show any lesion. The positive AFP with abdominal pain should still consider the possible diagnosis of liver cancer. He was explored by Dr. Zhaoyou Tang and Dr. Xinda Zhou in Sep 1987 at age 70 and diagnosis of liver cancer confirmed. The 6cm tumor was located in the left lateral lobe with a cancer thrombus in the left portal vein and extended into the main trunk. An En Bloc left hepatectomy with removal of the thrombus in the left branch and main trunk of the portal vein was performed. This procedure is usually considered palliative. In addition, silver clips were inserted into the portal area to guide post-op radiotherapy. Pathology confirmed HCC. Surprisingly, the prognosis was very good, by May 2015 at age 97, he was still alive and well with ongoing survival of 27 years.

Key Points to Remember

This was another case explored based on only a pre-op positive AFP and the cancer was successfully resected. We feel that for only AFP positive patients, exploration should be considered when they meet the following requirements: ① AFP > 400μg/L and persisted for more than 2 months, ② prior to operation, all modes of imaging studies if available, had been applied, such as: ultrasound, CT, MRI as well as hepatic angiography and ③ digestive tract and genital tumors excluded. At present, a variety of imaging studies are very advanced and sensitive. Any tumor exceeding 1cm is rarely missed. Therefore, patients with positive AFP but negative imaging studies should be followed-up closely.

Generally, a palliative resection is less effective than a radical resection, but this is not absolute. At times, a patient could achieve very good results after palliative resection. Mr. Li happened to be one of them. He was a HCC patient with cancer thrombus in the portal vein and had a satisfactory outcome. This could be due to the following: ① tumor and thrombus thoroughly removed, ② relatively good biologic characteristics of the tumor and ③ the patient had relatively good immune functions.

Improvement in survival rate is only our primary goal and increase of long-term survival is our highest goal. Of course, the ideal effect is not only to obtain long-term survival, but also a long life with high quality. Gratifyingly, certain liver cancer patients have realized their ideal goal and Mr. Li was one of them, He was the 2nd oldest patient (97 years old, the first was 99 in our series) and enjoyed happiness in his later life. Of course, the patient's longevity depended not only on successful treatment of liver cancer.

Case 51

(Admission No. 213809)
Two-Step Resection, Ongoing Survival 27 Years
（Nov 1987-   ）

Synopsis

Ms. Cheng, housewife, was born Jul 1938 in Yancheng, Jiangsu. She was referred to Zhongshan Hospital for upper abdominal discomfort, positive AFP (568μg/L) and a space-occupying lesion in the liver on type-B ultrasound. In Nov 1987 at age 49, exploration by Dr. Zenghen Ma and Dr. Weiping Yang revealed a tumor 7cm in the right lobe close to the 2nd hepatic hilum and inferior vena cava with mild liver cirrhosis. Diagnosis by needle biopsy was HCC. As she was diabetic and her tumor close to major vessels, forceful resection could carry great risks. It was decided to perform right hepatic artery ligation, right hepatic artery embolization with gelfoam, intra-tumor ethanol injection and insertion of silver clips around the tumor area to guide post-op external radiotherapy, 4,500r radiotherapy was given at the Shanghai Tumor Hospital. Surprisingly, the tumor dramatically shrank with significant decrease of AFP (568μg/L to normal). After 4 months, in Mar 1988, the

2nd operation was performed. The tumor had reduced to 3cm. A right partial resection was smoothly performed by Dr. Zhaoyou Tang and Dr. Zhengchen Ma and recovery satisfactory. The tumor specimen was hard in texture, capsule thick and with massive necrosis. Pathology was tumor necrosis with no viable tumor cell. Follow-up by May 2015 at age 76, she was well with ongoing survival of 27 years.

Other Relevant Data

She had hepatitis 12 years ago, but no family history of liver cancer.

She was treated with Traditional Chinese Medicine for a short time after the first operation. But after the 2nd operation no adjuvant treatment was given.

She was very cautious with her diet. She is one of those who believed that chicken and seafood could be carcinogenic. She never ate seafood or chicken. She liked to eat vegetables and fruits.

Key Points to Remember

This is a very successful case of the 2-step resection for liver cancer. The results are: ① the tumor shrank to 1/2 of the original size after the hepatic artery procedure, ② after the first operation AFP decreased to normal, ③ pathology of tumor specimen showed complete necrosis with no viable tumor cell and ④ 27 years with no recurrence or metastasis.

We feel there is no relationship between the good curative effect and her "restrictions on foods". Reasons for the good effect might be: ① the tumor was not very large, only 7 cm in size, ② application of comprehensive treatment such as hepatic artery surgery, ethanol injection and external radiotherapy and ③ less virulent biologic characteristics of the tumor.

How large a tumor is suitable for hepatic artery surgery? This problem cannot be generalized. We feel a huge or giant tumor that is not suitable for surgical resection, a hepatic artery procedure should be considered. When the tumor is not big, but near the hepatic hilum or with severe cirrhosis or the patient's general condition is relatively poor, a hepatic artery procedure should also be considered.

A hepatic artery procedure and its postoperative treatment is relatively complex. It is also not a panacea. It is not indicated in advanced and terminal liver cancer.

Case 52

(Admission N0. 215719)
A Single Resection, Ongoing Survival 27 Years
(Feb 1988-   )

Synopsis

Mr. Yan was from Henan. He had no history of hepatitis or family history of liver cancer. Due to positive AFP and a space-occupying lesion in the liver on type-B ultrasound and CT scan during cholecystitis follow-up, he was operated on in Feb 1988 at age 50. The tumor 10cm×5cm×5cm was in the right lobe (segments Ⅴ-Ⅵ-Ⅶ-Ⅷ) with mild cirrhosis. As the residual liver was adequate with no surgical contraindication, even though the tumor was big hepatic resection was decided. For safety, the incision was extended to become a thoracoabdominal incision. Subtotal hepatectomy of the right lobe was carried out successfully by Dr. Xinda Zhou and Dr. Yanming Bao. AFP returned from 56μg/L to normal. Pathology was grade Ⅱ-Ⅲ differentiated HCC. Follow-up by May 2015, he was still healthy with ongoing survival of 27 years.

Key Points to Remember

A large number of clinical data indicate that there is no close relationship between tumor size and AFP concentration. Do not mistakenly believe that lowly elevated AFP must be accompanied by small liver cancer. This patient is a typical case. Although his AFP was only 56μg/L, the tumor had reached 10cm in size. Therefore, comprehensive assessment and cumulative clinical experience contributed to improvement in therapeutic results in liver cancer.

At present, with the advent of new medical equipment and improved surgical skills, almost all liver resections are performed with a subcostal incision. The thoracoabdominal incision for liver operation has been abandoned.

Case 53

（Admission No. 222360）
A Single Resection, Ongoing Survival 27 Years
(Aug 1988-   )

Synopsis

Ms Wang, textile worker, was born Oct 1951 and worked in Shanghai. Due to dull right epigastric pain for 20 days, positive AFP and a space-occupying lesion in the liver on type-B ultrasound and CT scan, in Aug 1988 at age 37, she was explored. A tumor 9cm×6cm×4.5cm in the middle lobe of the liver (segments Ⅳ - Ⅴ, between the left medial and right anterior lobes), close to the gallbladder with several tiny satellite nodules was found. A partial middle hepatectomy and cholecystectomy were performed by Dr. Xinda Zhou and Dr. Zengchen Ma. Pathology was HCC. AFP dropped from 400μg/L to normal. Chinese Herbal Medicine was given for 2 years. Interferon injections and cisplatin, doxorubicin systemic chemotherapy administered for a short time. Her outcome was very satisfactory. Follow-up by Sep 2015 at 63, she was healthy with ongoing survival of 27 years.

Other Relevant Data

She had HBV infection in 1979. Her father died of unspecified liver disease. Her young brother died of liver cancer in 1985.

She had fracture of the left femoral neck and received surgery at Huashan Hospital.

She is optimistic and kind-hearted. She believed in modern medicine. She actively cooperated with her physicians. She is willing to share with other patients her anti-cancer experiences. She is a member of the Shanghai Club for Cancer Recovery and actively participated in relevant activities.

She has a wide range of food options including chicken, duck, mutton and sea food without any unusual dietary habits and restrictions.

She is very concerned about quality of life and enjoys happy life. One of her favorites is travel. She had been to many scenic spots in China, Australia, Russia and the Nordic countries.

Her mother and husband are in good health. Her son was 8 years old when she had her operation and is now married. The 3 generations live a happy life together.

Surgeon's Profile

Prof. Xinda Zhou was born 1939 in Zhejiang, a senior Hepatic Oncology Surgeon, Former Vice Chairman of the Liver Cancer Institute. He graduated from Shanghai First Medical College in 1963 and became a surgeon at Zhongshan Hospital.

Dr. Zhou has devoted his life to clinical research in hepatocellular carcinoma for more than 40 years. He had treated and cured a large number of liver cancer patients. He had published more then 400 articles including a number of reports on long-term survival of liver cancer. He and colleagues won the National First Prize Award for Progress in Science and Technology, P.R. China. He had made great contributions in liver cancer research.

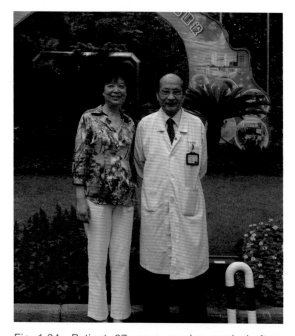

Fig. 1.34   Patient, 27 years ongoing survival after a single resection. Dr. Xinda Zhou and patient. (Sep 2015, in front of lawn in West Section of Zhongshan Hospital)

Key Points to Remember

Thus far, surgical resection is still the best treatment for liver cancer. The greatest advantage of surgery is its thoroughness. This patient's tumor was in the middle lobe of the liver, 9cm and with small satellite nodules. Complete resection of the tumor and satellite nodules achieved the best outcome in this case.

At present, local treatment of liver cancer is very popular. Radiofrequency ablation, microwave and anhydrous alcohol injection can sometimes produce a similar curative effect. But for large tumors more than 5cm, their efficacy is far from ideal.

Case 54

(Admission No. 224926)
A Single Resection, Total Survival 26 Years
(Nov 1988–Jan 2015)

Synopsis

Ms. Chen, housewife, was born Jan 1933 in Zhejiang, lived in Shanghai. She had no hepatitis history or family history of liver cancer. Due to right upper abdominal discomfort, positive AFP (>400μg/L) and a space-occupying lesion in the liver on type-B ultrasound and CT scan, she was explored by Dr. Zengchen Ma and Dr. Deting Zhan in Nov 1988 at age 55. Operation found 2 tumors, one large tumor 8cm×7.5cm×6cm in the right lower part of the liver (segment Ⅵ) and the other 2.5cm×2.5cm×2cm in the right upper part (segment Ⅷ) close to the 2nd hilum with no liver cirrhosis. Right partial hepatectomy was performed for the large tumor. For safety, 15ml anhydrous ethanol was injected into the small tumor instead of resection. The patient recovered well with no complications and her AFP dropped to normal. Pathology was moderately differentiated HCC. For 26 years (1988–2014) she lived a happy life with no recurrence or metastasis. Unfortunately, the patient died of senile dementia in Jan 2015 at age 82.

Other Relevant Data

Her son had severe cirrhosis and several episodes of upper gastrointestinal bleeding. In Dec 2007 at age 55, he received a liver transplantation at Zhongshan Hospital. Recovery was uneventful. Follow-up by May 2015, he had been living a quiet and happy life.

She was a devout Christian. She was frugal and kindhearted. She always cared about her fellow Christians, especially those who needed help.

Key Points to Remember

Almost all treatment modalities for liver cancer have advantages and disadvantages. We should tailor the treatment to meet the specific condition. In other words, we should not treat all HCC patients with only one modality. She had two liver cancer nodules, a small one near the inferior vena cava and a large one in the lower edge of the right liver. We achieved a good result in the treatment of the large tumor by resection and the small one by ethanol injection. It could be quite dangerous if both were resected. Alcohol injection is only used in small tumors.

Case 55

(Admission No. 230523)
Two-Step Resection, Ongoing Survival 26 Years
(Nov 1988-　)

Synopsis

Mr. Gou, was born in Nanchong, Sichuan. He had no history of hepatitis or family history of liver cancer. This is another 2-step resection case. The first operation was in Nov 1988 at age 49, at the Southwest Hospital in Chongqing, Sichuan. The tumor 10.5cm was located in the right postero-superior part of the liver close to the 2nd hepatic hilum with no liver cirrhosis. A simply right hepatic artery ligation with no catheterization was performed. After 8 months, the tumor reduced dramatically to 2.6cm in size and AFP dropped from 2,500μg/L to 73μg/L. The 2nd operation, right partial hepatectomy was performed by Dr. Zengchen Ma and Dr. Ming Zhang in Jul 1989 at Shanghai Zhongshan Hospital. Post-op recovery was uneventful and AFP returned to normal. Pathology was HCC with extensive necrosis. Follow-up by May 2015 at age 75, he was healthy with ongoing survival of 26 years.

Key Points to Remember

Hepatic artery surgery includes 3 procedures: hepatic artery ligation with hepatic artery catheterization, simply hepatic artery ligation and simply hepatic artery catheterization. In general, hepatic artery ligation is combined with catheterization, followed by intra-arterial chemotherapy. At times, adjuvant post-op irradiation therapy is administered to enhance therapeutic results.

At times, only a hepatic artery ligation is performed as dictated by the specific onsite situation. Generally, hepatic artery ligation alone is less effective than ligation with catheterization. Occasionally, ligation alone could also produce the desired effect. This case is one of them.

This case indicated that hepatic artery ligation is an important method in the treatment of liver cancer. At times, it is just as effective as resection or other treatment modalities.

Case 56

(Admission No. 245200)
A Single Resection, Ongoing Survival 24 Years
(Feb 1991−   )

Synopsis

Mr. Chen, was from Anhui. The patient had no hepatitis history or family history of liver cancer. He was referred to Zhongshan Hospital due to positive AFP and a space-occupying lesion on ultrasound and CT scan during check-up. In Feb 1991 at age 61, he was operated on by Dr. Yeqin Yu and Dr. Dongbo Xu. The tumor 2.5cm located in the right anterior lobe and a right partial hepatectomy was performed. AFP dropped from 384μg/L to normal. Pathology was HCC. Interferon injections and Chinese Herbal Medicine were given for 3 years. Follow-up by May 2015, he was 85 years old, still healthy with ongoing survival of 24 years.

Other Relevant Data

He is optimistic, believed in modern medicine and actively cooperated with his physicians.

He gave up smoking and drinking after surgery. He felt that chicken and seafood could be carcinogenic and avoided them. But he enjoyed beef and mutton.

He had a mild cerebral hemorrhage in 1980 but recovered with no sequelae.

Case 57

(Admission No. 246929)
Two-Step Resection and Resection of Recurrence, Ongoing Survival 24 Years
(Apr 1991－   )

Synopsis

Mr. Zhang, educator, was born Apr 1940 in Xinhui, Guangdong and worked in Shanghai. He had 3 kinds of malignant tumors in succession: malignant lymphoma of the head and neck, liver cancer and colon cancer. All were pathology confirmed.

Malignant lymphoma was diagnosed in 1965 at age 25. The submandibular, supraclavicular, axillary, inguinal and retroperitoneal lymph nodes were involved. Systemic chemotherapy and radiotherapy were given by Dr. Weiyu Tang at the Shanghai Tumor Hospital. He was completely cured in 1977.

His 2nd malignancy was liver cancer and received 3 operations. The first was in Apr 1991 at age 51. The tumor 20cm, size of a watermelon located in the right lobe of the liver with no cirrhosis. Diagnosis by needle biopsy was HCC. After careful assessment a right hepatic artery ligation and catheterization were carried out by Dr. Zhaoyou Tang and Dr. Yongshen Yuan. Epirubicin, cisplatin and ^{131}I-labeled anti-HCC monoclonal antibody beads were given intra-arterially by Dr. Shaochong Zeng. After 8 months, the tumor dramatically reduced to less than 10cm. In Dec 1991 a right partial hepatectomy was performed By Dr. Zhaoyou Tang and Dr. Zengchen Ma. Pathology was grade-II HCC. After 16 years, in Feb 2007, a 1cm recurrence in the left lateral lobe was detected and timely resected by Dr. Lunxiu Qin and Dr. Huichuan Sun.

The third malignancy was ascending colon cancer. In May 2010 at age 70, a right hemicolectomy was performed by Dr. Liqing Yao and Dr. Lujun Song. Pathology was adenocarcinoma of the colon with no lymphatic spread (0/8). No adjuvant treatment was administered.

Follow-up by Sep 2015 at age 75, he was alive and well, with no recurrence or metastasis from his liver cancer, colon cancer or malignant lymphoma. He survived 50 years after lymphoma treatment and 24 years after liver cancer resection.

Other Relevant Data

He had HBV hepatitis in 1977, but no family history of liver cancer.

His liver cancer was extremely huge (20cm), but AFP was negative (<20μg/L).

In addition to his 3 cancers, he also had other comorbidities.

He had had altogether 6 major operations in his lifetime.

Summary of the 3 malignancies and his 6 operations

In 1960 at age 20, the 1st operation was right pneumonectomy for tuberculosis at the Shanghai Second Tuberculosis Hospital.

In 1965–1977 at age 25–37, external radiotherapy and systemic chemotherapy for malignant lymphoma at the Shanghai Tumor Hospital.

In Apr 1991 at age 51, the 2nd operation or the 1st liver cancer operation, a right hepatic artery ligation and catheterization at Zhongshan Hospital.

In Dec 1991 at age 51, the 3rd operation or the 2nd liver cancer operation, a right partial hepatectomy at Zhongshan Hospital.

In May 2000 at age 60, the 4th operation was emergency cholecystectomy and choledocholithotomy for cholelithiasis by the Dept. of General Surgery, Zhongshan Hospital.

In Feb 2007 at age 67, the 5th operation or the 3rd liver cancer operation, a left lateral segmentectomy for recurrence at Zhongshan Hospital.

In May 2010 at age 70, the 6th operation, a right hemicolectomy for ascending colon cancer by the Dept. of General Surgery, Zhongshan Hospital.

Discussion

Life sometimes depended on luck or fate. Some have very good luck, never had any tumor. Others were less so and tumor occurred at a certain period of life. A few even had the worse luck and suffered from several tumors synchronously or metachronously. Treatment outcome sometimes is also linked to luck. With bad luck, early or even a small tumor did not necessarily yield good results. With good luck, even huge or multiple tumors, could have a good outcome with long-term survival. He was one of the latter. He suffered from 3 malignant tumors: malignant lymphoma, liver cancer and colon cancer. His luck was not good. But with surgery, comprehensive treatment and his tenacious perseverance in his struggle with tumors, he finally won and led a long life. It was a very unusual case. It reflected the progress in modern medicine and the strong will of the patient in his battle against cancer.

As mentioned before, the curative effect of a malignant tumor depended on many factors. For Mr. Zhang, in addition to modern medicine and technology, his mental status and personality also played an important role. We feel that the patient has the following characteristics: ① treating the disease with a materialistic attitude. Take things in their stride and face them boldly as they appear, with no anxiety or mental breakdown; ② believe in science, modern medicine and can actively cooperate with his physicians. Willing to bear the pains and costs, especially those of surgery, chemotherapy and radiotherapy; ③ being cheerful, optimistic, contended, easily satisfied and never being secluded or lonely, thereby avoided unnecessary troubles and a heavy mental burden; ④ paying attention to both treatment and work. As long as his disease was stable, and his physician allowed, he returned to work, but not overly stressed. He worked until retirement at age 60; ⑤ paying attention to work as well as rest, and avoid overworking; ⑥ has a wide-range of food options without any restrictions or unusual dietary whims.

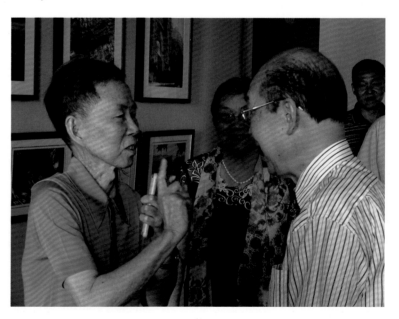

Fig. 1.35　24 years ongoing survival after two-step resection and resection of recurrence of liver cancer

Patient (left) and surgeon, Prof. Zhaoyou Tang (right) in Aug 2015 in Dr. Tang's office

Key Points to Remember

This is a very unfortunate patient. He had 3 kinds of malignant tumors and two of them were very serious and complicated.

This was also a case of successful treatment of malignant tumors. The 3 tumors were basically cured. There was ongoing survival of 50 years for malignant lymphoma and 24 years for liver cancer.

This is an example of successful comprehensive treatment of malignant tumors: combination of radiotherapy and chemotherapy for malignant lymphoma as well as combination of hepatic artery ligation and intra-arterial chemotherapy for liver cancer.

The success of these treatments indicated that a hepatic artery operation is very effective in the treatment of large HCC. It can reduce tumor size, lead to necrosis, prolong life and create opportunities for the 2-step resection. The 2-step resection is superior to immediate resection when the liver cancer is huge.

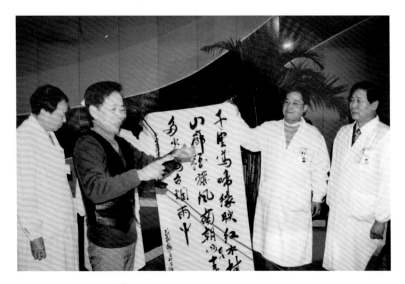

Fig. 1.36   Patient (2nd, left) reciting poem "Spring in Jiangnan". Patient loved calligraphy and ancient Chinese poetry. In the "Heart to Heart Activity"at the 30th Anniversary of the establishment of the Liver Cancer Institute in Dec 1999, he wrote down the poem "Spring in Jiangnan" by a Tang Dynasty poet on the spot. He wished the Liver Cancer Institute could be like "Spring in the South", like in the lower reaches of the Yangtze River, full of vitality, achieving great progress in liver cancer research and he thanked the hard work of the medical staff of Zhongshan Hospital

Dr. Zhiquan Wu (1st, left), Dr. Jin Zhou (2nd, right) and Dr. Zengchen Ma (1st, right)

This is also an example of successful treatment with physician-patient co-operation. The patient believed in modern medicine and actively cooperated with his physicians to make the implementation of treatment possible. On the other hand, the physician after full assessment of the situation, strategically formulated the optimal plan of action.

Case 58

(Admission No. 252677)
Resection of Bilateral Lesions, Ongoing Survival 23 Years
(Dec 1991–   )

Synopsis

Mr. Huang, physician, was born Sep 1938 in Ningbo, Zhejiang and worked in Shanghai. In 1989, He sought medical care due to fatigue, type-B ultrasound found a space-occupying lesion in the liver. He was not further investigated because his AFP was negative. In Dec 1991 at age 53, he came to Zhongshan Hospital and was diagnosed to have liver cancer according to the characteristics on type-B ultrasound and CT scan. Exploration found 2 lesions, a bigger one 4cm in the right anterior lobe of the liver and a smaller one 2cm in the left lateral lobe. Right and left lateral partial hepatectomies were performed by Dr. Zengchen Ma and Dr. Yaxin Zheng. As strongly requested by the patient's wife, the abdominal cavity was irrigated with 1,000mg fluorouracil in normal saline before closure. Pathology was HCC. Post-op. TACE was performed and Chinese Herbal Medicine given for 5 years. Follow-up by Sep 2015 at age 77, he remained healthy with ongoing survival of 23 years.

Other Relevant Data

The patient had nonicteric hepatitis in 1978. His elder brother died of liver cancer.

The patient had a positive attitude of life and was kind-hearted. He believed in modern science and led a normal life. He had no special habits or food selections.

Key Points to Remember

It is not a routine to lavage the abdominal cavity with anticancer drugs before closure in liver cancer operations. We feel that the importance of a no-touch technique can never be over emphasized in tumor surgery. In order to avoid recurrence and improve outcome, the ligaments around the liver should be thoroughly sectioned to mobilize the liver and the surgeons should minimize and avoid directly touching the tumor.

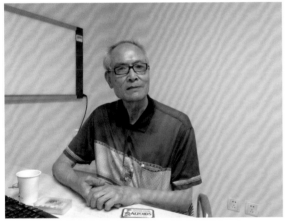

Fig. 1.37   Patient, 23 years ongoing survival after resection.(Aug 2015 at Outpatient Clinic of Zhongshan Hospital)

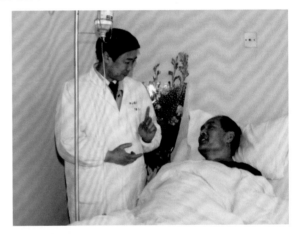

Fig. 1.38   Dr. Zengchen Ma at P.O visit on day 9, Dec 1991

Case 59

(Admission No. 253002)
Liver Resection and Hepatic Vein Cancer Thrombectomy,
Ongoing Survival 23 Years
(Dec 1991‾   )

Synopsis

Mr. Ma was born Jun 1954 in Shanghai and worked in Dujun, Guizhou

He had upper abdominal discomfort, positive AFP and a space-occupying lesion in the liver on type-B ultrasound and CT scanning. In Dec 1991 at age 37, he was explored at Zhongshan Hospital. The huge tumor 15cm was in the left lateral lobe with a tumor thrombus, 2cm×1cm, in the left hepatic vein and extended into the inferior vena cava. An En Bloc resection including the left lateral lobe as well as left hepatic vein and thrombus was performed by Dr. Zengchen Ma and Dr. Binhong Yu. Pathology was HCC. The operation was difficult, but he recovered well. AFP dropped from 2,574µg/L to normal. As the tumor was huge and with a thrombus, he received 3 arterial chemoembolization at a hospital in Guizhou after discharge and TCM therapy was given for half a year. Follow-up by Sep 2015 at age 61, he remained healthy with ongoing survival of 23 years.

Other Relevant Data

The patient had no hepatitis history, but a family history of hepatic disease and liver cancer. His mother died of cirrhosis. His elder brother was found to have liver cancer after him, but was too late to be salvaged.

He had an open mind and believed in modern medicine. He cooperated well with his physicians.

He had a wide range of food options without any restrictions or peculiar dietary whims.

He did not give up drinking. At times, he still took a small amount of alcohol to relieve fatigue.

He and his wife both are now well and healthy. His son (10 years old when he was operated on), a university graduate has an ideal job and is married. The whole family is in happiness.

Key Points to Remember

This is the 3rd long-term survivor after En Bloc resection including the left lateral lobe with a huge cancer as well as removal of a tumor thrombus in the left hepatic vein. We feel that: ① huge liver cancer complicated with tumor thrombus in the left hepatic vein is not rare; ② at times, En Bloc resection of the cancer with removal of the thrombus in the left hepatic vein could yield a good outcome; ③ the operation has certain risks, we should avoid massive bleeding and air embolism during the procedure.

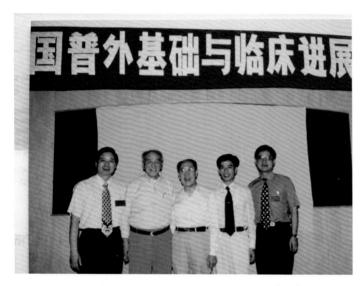

Fig. 1.39 Surgeons of the patient，Dr. Zengchen Ma (1st, left) and Dr. Jian Zhou (1st, right) together with fellow surgeons, Prof. Mengchao Wu (middle), Prof. Ruitu Ran (2nd, left) and Prof. Jiamei Yang (2nd, right), at a Surgical Conference. (Dec 1997 at Hainan)

Case 60

(Admission No. 253245)
A Single Resection, Ongoing Survival 23 Years
(Jan 1992-   )

Synopsis

Ms. Chen, physician, was born Apr 1949 in Shaoxing, Zhejiang and worked in Shanghai. She was found to have positive AFP and a space-occupying lesion in the liver on type-B ultrasound and CT scan during check-up. She received transcatheter arterial chemoembolization

(TACE) at the Dept of Interventional Radiology, Zhongshan Hospital on Jan 3 1992，because no surgical bed was available. On Jan 27 1992 at age 43, she was explored by Dr. Zengchen Ma and Dr. Binhong Yu of the Dept. of Surgical Hepatic Oncology. The 3cm tumor located in the right lobe of the liver close to the gallbladder. A right partial hepatectomy as well as cholecystectomy was smoothly performed. Pathology was HCC with extensive necrosis. AFP decreased from 1,144μg/L to normal. No adjuvant therapy was given. Follow-up by Sep 2015 at age 66, the patient remained well with ongoing survival of 23 years.

Other Relevant Data

She had HBV hepatitis in 1976, but no family history of liver cancer.

She had a heart valve replacement in Apr 2014 by Dr. Chunsheng Wang at the Dept. of Cardiac Surgery, Zhongshan Hospital and convalescence was uneventful with satisfactory outcome.

After her cardiac surgery, she recovered well and was able to take part in social activities.

She had a wide range of food options with no special dietary preferences or restrictions.

Her husband is well and healthy. Her daughter (15 years old when she had her liver operation) is now a teacher, married and the mother of a lovely girl. The whole family, 3 generations are well and living a happy life.

Key Points to Remember

TACE could lead to necrosis of tumor, reduce tumor cell viability and improve surgery's effectiveness. This patient had a small HCC and a very good outcome after TACE. We feel pre-op TACE is not a routine. At times, it would delay the optimal time for surgical resection. We feel for huge liver cancers, those with no clear margin or with satellite nodules pre-op TACE could be considered.

Case 61

(Admission No. 257592)
A Single Resection, Ongoing Survival 23 Years
(Jun1992-   )

Synopsis

Mr. Yang was born Nov 1949, in Wuxi, Jiangsu. He was referred to Shanghai Zhongshan Hospital and explored in Jun 1992 at age 42, for dull right upper abdominal pain of 3 months, positive AFP and a small space-occupying lesion in the liver on type-B ultrasound and CT scanning. The tumor 2.8cm was located in the right postero-inferior part of the liver (segment Ⅵ) with no obvious cirrhosis. A right partial hepatectomy was performed by Dr. Zengchen Ma, and Dr. Jingen Zhang. Pathology was HCC. AFP returned from 455μg/L to normal. Interferon was given for 6 months and also Traditional Chinese Medicine. During the past 5 years, lamivudine and adefovir were given for an elevated HBV index. Follow-up by Sep 2015 at age 65, he was well with ongoing survival of 23 years.

Other Relevant Data

He had neither HBV hepatitis nor family history of liver cancer.

He liked to eat a variety of nutritious foods, such as seafood, beef, mutton and eggs except chicken. He felt chicken could be carcinogenic.

He had a few special eating habits. After operation, he took soy-bean milk with honey for 23 years. In addition, he ate ginger preserved in vinegar, soy sauce and crystal sugar every morning for 11 years.

His wife, daughter, son and 2 grandchildren are healthy and live happily together.

Personal Hobby

His favorite hobby was raising homing pigeons and took part in competitions. He had won many awards. The highest award was a

Second Prize in the National Pigeon Competition (Zhengzhou, Henan to Wuxi, Jiangsu, 700km) in 2000. He also won the Champion in another pigeon competition (Xi'an, Shaanxi to Wuxi, Jiangsu, 1000km). Regretfully, he had to give up his hobby after he moved to a new home in 2012. Pigeon raising was not allowed there.

Case 62

(Admission No. 257894)
A Single Resection, Ongoing Survival 23Years
(Jul 1992–   )

Synopsis

Mr. Chen, cadre of Shanghai Navigation Department, was born Mar 1955 in Shanghai. He was admitted for a 2.5cm space-occupying lesion in the liver on type-B ultrasound and CT scanning during check-up. The tumor was in the right lobe. In Jul 1992 at age 37, he was explored. Liver cancer confirmed and a right partial hepatectomy was smoothly performed by Dr. Zhengchen Ma and Dr. Mengle Xing. Pathology was moderately differentiated HCC. Traditional Chinese Medicine was given for 10 years and interferon for 3 years. He returned to work one year after operation Follow-up by Sep 2015 at age 60, he was well and healthy with ongoing survival of 23 years.

Other Relevant Data

He had no HBV hepatitis history, but a family history of liver cancer. His young brother died of liver cancer. Even more unfortunately, his mother also had liver cancer and was too late to be salvaged and passed away in 1994.

His wife is healthy. His son (6 years old when he was operated on) is married in 2012 and leads a happy life.

His AFP was only mildly positive. It returned from 97μg/L. to normal after operation.

His life was well regulated. He had no restrictions on foods, but liked light and delicate flavors. He did not like chicken or seafood.

He is now retired and often rides his motorcycle to go shopping. He also helps his wife with housework.

A way to keep in good health

He believed that massaging acupuncture points on the ear is beneficial. He learned "Auricular Massage" from a barefoot doctor in his unit. These acupuncture points on the ears, are mini replicas that reflect the functions of the organs and systems distributed throughout the body. Ear massage has the same effect as stimulating the corresponding points on the torso.

He not only believed and was keen on auricular massage. He also bought books and an auricular points model for study.

He felt right ear massage was more effective.

He believed ear massages could not only protect the liver, prevent and treat recurrence of liver cancer. It could also be useful in the prevention and treatment of other ailments, such as colds and respiratory diseases.

Key Points to Remember

HCC is either AFP positive or AFP negative. According to AFP concentration levels, patients with positive AFP can arbitrarily be categorized as: lowly elevated AFP (>20–200μg/L), moderate AFP (>200–10,000μg/L) and high AFP (>10,000μg/L). His AFP was 97μg/L, belonging to the AFP-lowly elevated HCC subgroup. According to our data, HCC patients with a lowly elevated AFP were not infrequent. He was the 5th liver cancer case with lowly elevated AFP. The others were case 25 (AFP 26μg/L), case 27 (50μg/L), case 31 (110μg/L) and case 52 (56μg/L) in our series. We feel that AFP concentration level has no relationship with tumor size and prognosis. In case 25 for example, the tumor was 16 cm, but AFP only 26μg/L.

As for the value of "ear acupoints massage", we have no experience and cannot make any comment. However, it apparently could do no harm and, if wished by the patient, might be used as a form of self-applied supplementary treatment.

Case 63

(Admission No. 261886)
A Single Resection, Total Survival 22 Years
(Dec 1992–Apr 2015)

Synopsis

Mr. He, township cadre, was born Oct 1933 in Ningbo, Zhejiang. He was referred to Shanghai Zhongshan Hospital for positive AFP and a 5cm space-occupying lesion in the right anterior lobe of the liver (segment Ⅴ) close to the gallbladder on type-B ultrasound and CT during check-up. In Dec 1992 at age 59, a right partial hepatectomy with cholecystectomy was performed by Dr. Zengchen Ma and Dr. Xiaomin Wang. Pathology was HCC. AFP dropped from 392μg/L to normal. Chinese Herbal Medicine was given for 3 years. For 22 years, no recurrence or metastasis was detected on type-B ultrasound, CT scan and chest X-ray on regular check-up. Unfortunately, he also had multiple comorbidities: diabetes, hypertension, benign prostate hypertrophy. In Apr 2015 at age 81, he passed away due to cerebral apoplexy and multiple organ failure.

Other Relevant Data

He had HBV hepatitis in 1989, but no family history of liver cancer.

He had a wide range of food options (including chicken and red meat) with no restrictions. He was born and brought up in a costal city and had a natural predilection for seafood. Although he liked chicken, he gave it up after the bird flu epidemic.

Being a retired cadre, he remained politically alert, always kept himself updated on major events in the world and attended relevant meetings regularly.

Case 64

(Admission No. 262428)
A Single Resection, Ongoing Survival 22 Years
(Dec 1992–   )

Synopsis

Ms. He, garment factory worker, was born Mar 1951 in Shanghai. She was explored at Zhongshan Hospital for positive AFP and a space-occupying lesion in the liver on type-B ultrasound and CT during check-up. The tumor 3.5cm was located in the left lateral lobe of the liver with moderate cirrhosis. A left lateral segmentectomy was performed by Dr. Zengchen Ma and Dr. Shuqun Cheng in Dec 1992 at age 41. Pathology was HCC. The procedure was smooth and convalescence uneventful. Thymic peptide injection was given for 1 year and interferon for 3 months. She had annual regular check-ups and no recurrence or metastasis was detected. Follow-up by Sep 2015 at age 64, she was alive and well with ongoing survival of 22 years.

Other Relevant Data

She had HBV hepatitis in 1976 and a family history of hepatic cirrhosis and liver cancer. Her mother and uncle both died of massive upper gastrointestinal bleeding due to rupture of esophageal and fundal varices. Her 2 elder brothers and 1 young sister all died of liver cancer.

She was AFP positive. After operation AFP returned from 2,037μg/L to normal.

She had no restrictions on foods, but did not like chicken and red meat.

Believe it or not

She was asymptomatic. She recalled that she went to a check-up on her son's urge. He (then only 6 years old) dreamed she had liver cancer. We feel this could merely be a coincidence. As too many in the family had liver cancer, it created a deep impression on the mind of the young child and dreamed his mother was suffering from liver cancer.

Key Points to Remember

According to our data, it is not uncommon for a family to have many members suffering from liver cancer. Case 42 is the most typical. Among siblings 5 of 7 suffered from liver cancer. Luckily, 3 were cured by surgery. It is not very clear, what made a family have many liver cancers. Some think it is genetic, others think it is mother-child transmission and still others believe that it is due to the common living conditions in a poor environment or unhealthy eating habits in the family.

The good news is that there is a decreasing incidence in liver cancer. This may be related to improvement in the living environment, changes in diet habits and the wide application of hepatitis B vaccination.

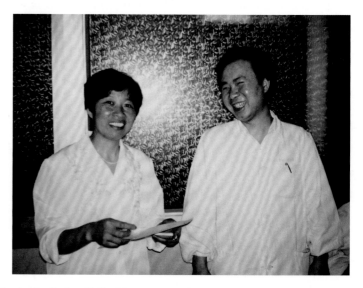

Fig. 1.40   Patient(left), 22 years ongoing survival after a single resection. Photo taken the 3rd year (Jun 1995) after resection

Case 65

(Admission No. 264053)
Liver Resection for Metastases from Colon Cancer, Ongoing
Survival 22 Years
(Mar 1993–   )

Synopsis

Mr. Gao, cadre, was born Sep 1939 in Cixi, Zhejiang and worked in Shanghai. This is a colon cancer case with metachronous liver metastases. The patient has a long-term survival after two surgeries.

His first operation, a partial colectomy was performed for descending colon cancer by Dr. Enchong Tang in Sep 1991 at Shanghai Renji Hospital. Systemic chemotherapy was given for 1 year and interferon 1/2 year. In Feb 1993, a solid space-occupying lesion was detected on type-B ultrasound and CT and diagnosed as liver metastasis from the colon cancer. In Mar 1993 at age 53, he had his second operation. Two tumors in the liver were found, one 2cm in the middle hepatic lobe close to the gallbladder and the other 2.5cm in the right lobe. There was no cirrhosis. Two partial hepatectomies with cholecystectomy were carried out by Dr. Zengchen Ma and Dr. Xiaomin Wang. The procedure was smooth and convalescence satisfactory. Chinese Herbal Medicine was administered for 8 years with no other adjuvant treatment. Pathology was metastatic adenocarcinoma. Follow-up by Sep 2015 at age 76, he was alive and well with ongoing survival of 22 years after the liver resection.

Other Relevant Data

In Jul 2010, he had a cerebral infarction but fortunately almost completely recovered with only mild sequelae. He could still go travelling (Shanghai to Beijing).

This patient had no family history of colon cancer, but had a family history of liver diseases. His father died of end stage cirrhosis and elder brother of primary liver cancer.

He had a wide range of food options with no restrictions. He liked sea food, did not drink but smoked. He felt drinking was harmful.

His wife, 2 sons and 2 granddaughters are healthy and live happily together.

Key Points to Remember

Liver cancer can be divided into two types: primary and secondary. In Western countries, secondary liver cancer is more common. Whereas, in China primary liver cancer is more common. Secondary liver cancer is mostly from colorectal cancer.

Liver resection and certain regional therapies still are the most effective for secondary liver cancer.

We feel systemic chemotherapy after liver resection in secondary liver cancer is not necessary. The 3 cases (including this one) in our series all survived more than 20 years after hepatectomy.

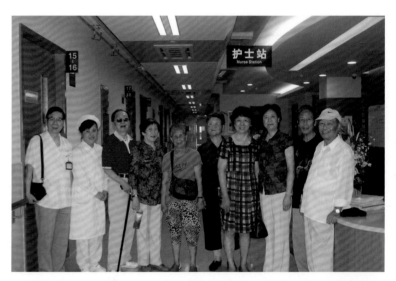

Fig. 1.41　Patient (3rd, left, in red T-shirt) 22 years ongoing survival after liver resection for metastases from colon cancer and other long-term survivors visiting new ward of the Dept. of Surgical Hepatic Oncology, Zhongshan Hospital in Aug 2015

Case 66

(Admission No. 264421)
Resection of Hepatic Hilum Cancer, Ongoing Survival 22
Years
(Mar 1993‒   )

Synopsis

Mr. Ye, cadre, was born Jun 1944 in Quzhou, Zhejiang. He sought medical care for a cold, but type-B ultrasound and CT both showed a space-occupying lesion in the liver. His AFP was negative (12μg/L). He was referred to Shanghai Zhongshan Hospital and a possible primary liver cancer was suspected. In Mar 1993 at age 48, he was explored. A tumor 6.5cm was located in the right antero-superior part of the liver (segment Ⅷ) close to the second hepatic hilum. The tumor was sandwiched between the middle, right hepatic veins and inferior vena cava.

Although it was a difficult case, it was still decided to perform a right partial hepatectomy. The second hepatic hilum where the right and middle hepatic veins joined the inferior vena cava was carefully isolated and protected. To control bleeding, intermittent hepatic artery and portal vein (hepato-duodenal ligament) occlusion (Pringle maneuver) was also applied (4 times, a total of 31 minutes). The tumor was completely, safely removed by Dr. Zengchen Ma and Dr. Xiaomin Wang. Pathology was HCC. Systemic chemotherapy was given for 10 days and discontinued duo to hair loss. Interferon was given for 1 year. Follow-up by Sep 2015 at age 71, he was alive with ongoing survival of 22 years.

Other Relevant Data

He had HBV hepatitis in 1974, but no family history of liver cancer.

A year after operation, his AFP fluctuated for a time, rising as high as 2,000μg/L. It was considered the result of liver regeneration rather than tumor recurrence or metastasis, as no recurrence or metastasis was detected on imaging examinations. After supportive treatment, liver function and AFP both returned to normal.

In addition to liver cancer surgery, he also had two other operations. In Dec 2007, he underwent cholecystectomy for cholelithiasis at Zhongshan Hospital and lithotripsy for left renal calculi in 2013.

His life was well regulated, getting up at 8 AM and going to bed at 11 PM. He also took a walk every day.

He had a wide range of food options (including chicken, red meat and seafood) and had no special eating habits or restrictions. He gave up smoking and drinking after liver resection.

He is a very kind-hearted and optimistic person and has a positive attitude of life. He shared with other patients his anticancer experiences without any reserve.

He funded 8 young persons to go to college as a token repaying society and thank the medical staff that gave him a second life and all those that took care of him.

Key Points to Remember

Liver cancer at the hepatic hilum refers to those located less than 1 cm from the first, second or third hepatic hilum. Liver cancer at the hepatic hilum is not uncommon. Liver cancer at the hepatic hilum

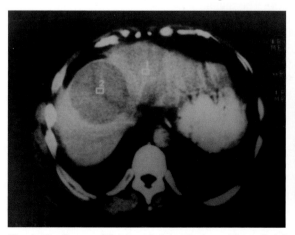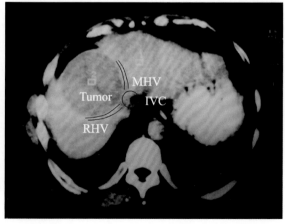

Fig. 1.42　Pre-op CT scan showing lesion at hepatic hilum. left: Original scan, right: CT scan with label depicting tumor, inferior vena cava, middle hepatic vein and right hepatic vein

is not contraindicated to liver resection. With protection of the large vessels and large bile ducts and if necessary, intermittent occlusion of first hepatic hilum, cancer at the hepatic hilum could be completely and safely resected. A good or even excellent outcome could be obtained if surgeon paid special attention to the no-touch tumor technique, avoid and reduce squeezing of the tumor when operating.

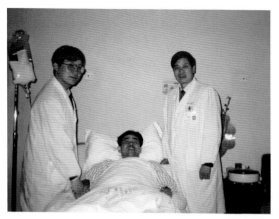

Fig. 1.43   Patient and his surgeons, Dr. Zengchen Ma (right), Dr. Shuangjian Qiu on the 7th post-op day (Mar 1993)

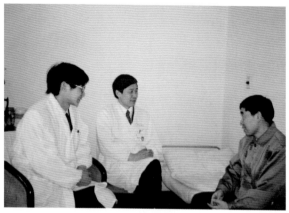

Fig. 1.44   Dr. Zengchen Ma (surgeon, middle), Dr. Jinglin Xia (internist, left) and patient discussing future treatment Apr 1994

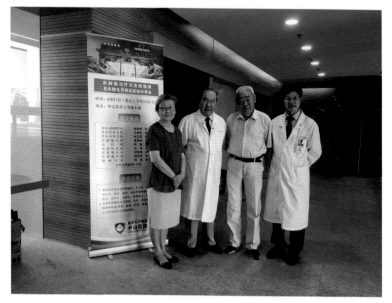

Fig. 1.45   Patient (2nd, right) and internists, Prof. Zhiyin Lin (1st, left), Prof. Binghui Yang (2nd, left) and Prof. Jinglin Xia(1st, right), 22 years ongoing survival after a single resection of hepatic hilum cancer

Case 67

(Admission No. 265206)
A Single Resection, Ongoing Survival 22 Years
(Apr 1993–   )

Synopsis

Mr. Jiang was born Feb 1954 in Shanghai. He sought medical care for chronic cholecystitis, but Type-B ultrasound and CT both showed a space-occupying lesion in the liver. With positive AFP, he was referred to Zhongshan Hospital. A tumor 3.5cm was located in the right posterior lobe (segment VII) with no cirrhosis. A right partial hepatectomy was smoothly performed at age 39 by Dr. Zengchen Ma and Dr. Xiaomin Wang in Apr 1993. Pathology was moderately differentiated HCC. AFP decreased from 2,241µg/L to normal. Chinese Herbal Medicine was given for 8 years and interferon for 3 months. Follow-up by Sep 2015 at age 61, he was well with ongoing survival of 22 years.

Other Relevant Data

He had HBV hepatitis in 1971, but no family history of liver cancer.

He is optimistic and cheerful. His life was well regulated and had no particular hobby.

He had no special food restrictions, but did not like crab meat.

His wife is in good health. His son was 4 years old when he had his operation. Now the boy is a graduate of a famous university, has an ideal job and preparing to get married at the end of 2015.

Case 68

(Admission No. 265765)
A Single Resection, Ongoing Survival 22 Years
（May 1993-   ）

Synopsis

Mr. Gao, judge, was born Dec 1945 in Jinan, Shandong and worked in Hanzhong, Shaanxi. He was referred to Shanghai Zhongshan Hospital for right upper abdominal discomfort of one month and a space-occupying lesion in the liver on type-B ultrasound and CT with positive AFP. A tumor 3.5cm was located in the middle lobe of the liver with no cirrhosis. A partial middle hepatectomy was carried out at age 47 by Dr. Zengchen Ma and Dr. Xiaomin Wang in May 1993. The procedure was smooth and convalescence uneventful. Systemic chemotherapy, interferon and Chinese Herbal medicine were given for a short period and discontinued duo to adverse effects. Pathology was grade- Ⅱ HCC. AFP returned from 2,463μg/L to normal. Since 2009, he also has mild controlled hypertension and diabetes. No recurrence or metastasis was detected on type-B ultrasound, CT and chest X-ray on regular check-ups. Follow-up by May 2015 at age 69, he was in good health with ongoing survival of 22 years.

Other Relevant Data

He had no HBV hepatitis or family history of liver cancer.

He had a wide range of food options and liked fresh water fish.

He shared willingly with other patients his anticancer experiences without any reserve.

He retired in 2006. His life is well regulated, getting up at 7 AM and going to bed at 10 PM.

He did exercise by taking walk and biking every day, at the same time, buying vegetables on the way.

He also helps his wife with housework.

His wife is in good health. He has a son and a daughter, age 23 and 20, respectively when he was being operated. Now they are all married and have their own children. The 3 generations are all well and living a happy life.

Case 69

(Admission No. 22707)
A Single Resection in an 18 Months Child, Ongoing Survival 22 Years
(May 1993–   )

Synopsis

This little girl was born Nov 1991 in East China, referred to Shanghai Zhongshan Hospital due to a mass in the abdomen. Type-B ultrasound and CT showed a space-occupying lesion in the liver with positive AFP. A possible liver cancer was suspected. She was operated on by surgeons jointly from the Zhongshan Hospital and the SMU Affiliated Children's Hospital in May 1993 at age 18 months. An encapsulated tumor 8 cm was located in the right inferior lobe near the gallbladder. Texture of the liver was soft with no cirrhosis. A right partial hepatectomy with cholecystectomy was smoothly completed by Dr. Zengchen Ma and Dr. Xianmin Xiao. Convalescence was satisfactory. Pathology was HCC. AFP decreased from over 400μg/L to normal. No adjuvant treatment was given. Follow-up by Sep 2015 at age 23, she was in good health with ongoing survival of 22 years.

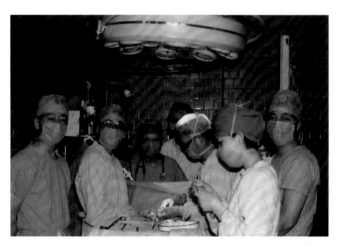

Fig. 1.46 An 18 months child, 22 years ongoing survival after a single resection. The girl being treated jointly by surgeons from Zhongshan Hospital and the SMU Affiliated Children's Hospital in May 1993

Other Relevant Data

She had no hepatitis history or family history of liver cancer.

She was a full term normal parturition baby.

Her parents did not accept further treatment because of financial difficulties.

Her parents and one elder brother are all in good health.

Her subsequent growth and development are entirely normal, not any different from other children.

She is now a university graduate and has a satisfactory job. She is also preparing to get married.

Key Points to Remember

Primary liver cancer often occurs in adults around age 50, but it is not rare in children or the aged. Radical resection is still the best treatment for patients with large HCC (> 5cm) whether in adults or children.

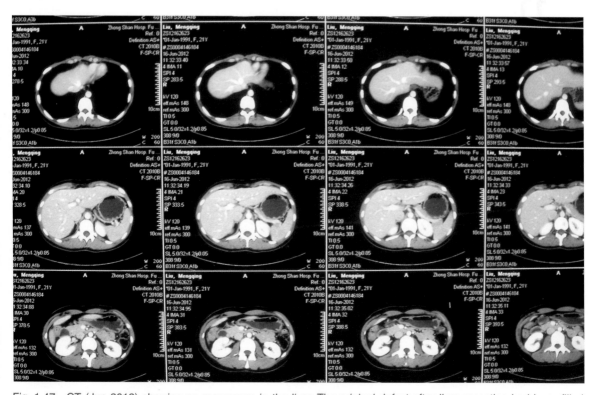

Fig. 1.47   CT (Jun 2012) showing no recurrence in the liver. The original defect after liver resection had been filled with newly generated liver

Case 70

(Admission No.268905)
A Single Resection, Ongoing Survival 22 Years
(Sep 1993−   )

Synopsis

Ms. Chen, worker, was born Mar 1964 in Liyang, Jiangsu. She sought medical care for a left upper abdominal mass and was referred to Shanghai Zhongshan Hospital. Type B ultrasound and CT both showed a space-occupying lesion in the liver. Although her AFP was normal (6μg/L), a possible primary liver cancer was still suspected. In Sep 1993 at age 29, she was explored. A tumor 7 cm was located in the left lateral lobe of the liver with no cirrhosis. An extended left lateral segmentectomy was smoothly performed by Dr. Zengchen Ma and Dr. Xuesheng Feng with uneventful convalescence. Thirty-doses of Interferon were given. Pathology was grade Ⅰ − Ⅱ HCC. Follow-up by Sep 2015 at age 51, she was in good health with ongoing survival of 22 years.

Other Relevant Data

She had no hepatitis history or family history of liver cancer.

She still worked as a shop assistant after resection.

She is an optimistic person with a positive attitude on life.

She has a wide range of food options (including chicken, red meat and seafood) with no special unusual eating habits.

Her husband is in good health. Her daughter (5 years old when she was operated on) is married and mother of 2 lovely sons. She is the youngest grandmother in our series and had her first grandchild when she was 45 years old (the 16th post-op year in 2009). The 3 generations are now well and living a happy life.

Case 71

(Admission No. 269338)
A Single Resection, Ongoing Survival 22 Years
(Sep 1993-)

Synopsis

Mr. Chen, manager of a grassroots enterprise, was born Nov 1954 in Zhenjiang, Jiangsu and worked in Suzhou. He sought medical care for a dull right upper abdominal pain. Type-B ultrasound and CT showed a space-occupying lesion in the liver. His AFP was normal. A possible primary liver cancer was suspected. A single tumor 4.5cm was located in the right postero-inferior part of the liver (segment Ⅵ) with mild liver cirrhosis. A right partial hepatectomy was smoothly performed by Dr. Zengchen Ma and Dr. Xuecheng Wang in Sep 1993. Interferon was given for 1 year. Pathology was HCC. Follow-up by Sep 2015 at age 60, he was in good health with ongoing survival of 22 years.

Other Relevant Data

He had no HBV hepatitis history or family history of liver cancer.

He was AFP negative, pre-op only 6µg/L.

In Nov 2013, he had a laparoscopic cholecystectomy for cholelithiasis at the Gulou Hospital in Nanjing. Both operation and convalescence were uneventful.

He felt a good mentality was very important in consolidating the surgical outcome of liver cancer. His experience was a liver cancer patient should not overwork and also avoid fatigue as well as mental burden.

Shortly after surgery, he returned to work.

He had no special unusual eating habits, occasionally smoked but did not drink.

He wrote many articles on diagnosis and treatment of liver cancer and tried to share his anticancer experiences with others, but unfortunately elicited no response.

Case 72

(Admission No. 270024)
Liver Resection for Metastasis from Colon Cancer, Total
Survival 21 Years
(Oct 1993–Feb 2015)

Synopsis

Mr. Li, civil servant, was born Jan 1935 in Taizhou, Jiangsu and worked in Shanghai. This is another metachronous liver metastasis in colon cancer with a long-term survival after 2 resections. His first operation was a partial colectomy for sigmoid colon cancer in Mar 1991 at the Shanghai Ruijin Hospital. Systemic and intra-abdominal chemotherapy as well as external radiation therapy were given post-op. In Sep 1993, type-B ultrasound and CT showed a space-occupying lesion in the liver with elevated CEA during follow-up. Liver metastasis from the colon cancer was suspected. The 2nd operation was performed Oct 1993 at age 58 at Zhongshan Hospital. A single 6cm tumor located in the left lateral lobe of the liver (segment Ⅱ) with no liver cirrhosis. A left lateral segmentectomy was performed by Dr. Zengchen Ma and Dr. Xuecheng Wang. Pathology was moderately differentiated metastatic adenocarcinoma with extensive necrosis. His CEA decreased from > 80ng/ml to normal. Chinese Herbal Medicine was given for 10 years. No recurrence or metastasis was found during annual check-up. Unfortunately, he died of uncontrolled diabetes in Feb 2015 at age 82. He survived 21 years after the liver resection.

Other Relevant Data

He had no hepatitis history or family history of liver cancer or colon cancer.

He was AFP negative (only 2μg/L).

He had a 3rd operation, cystectomy for bladder cancer in 2003 at the Shanghai Ruijin Hospital (Branch Division). Convalescence was uneventful and outcome satisfactory.

His diabetes was uncontrolled with gangrene of the right foot, which had to be amputated in Jan 2015. He died 20 days later.

Key Points to Remember

AFP is a marker of primary liver cancer, and CEA that of colorectal cancer. CEA is not as sensitive and specific as AFP. CEA is an important indicator of the existence of colorectal cancer and is used to monitor effectiveness of its treatment.

This is the 2nd long term survivor in our series after 2 operations for colon cancer and metachronous liver metastasis.

We feel colorectal cancer with liver metastasis (synchronous or metachronous) is not a terminal disease. An ideal outcome could still be achieved if effective treatment were implemented in time.

According to our data, systemic chemotherapy is not necessary for long-term survival of primary or secondary liver cancer.

Though this patient died of uncontrolled diabetic complications, we still have reason to believe that he was a lucky man: ① The patient overcame two cancers (colon cancer and bladder cancer), underwent 3 operations (a colectomy, a hepatectomy and a cystectomy) and achieved good outcomes. ② The patient's life expectancy was longer than the average of 74 years for Chinese males (WHO Report, 2005). ③ In 2008, his great-grandson was born and they lived a happy life "four generations under the same roof".

Case 73

(Admission No. 270917)
A Single Resection, Ongoing Survival 21 Years
(Nov 1993-   )

Synopsis

Mr. Shang, trade union cadre, was born Apr 1950 in Hangzhou and worked in Taizhou, Zhejiang. He was found to have positive AFP and a space-occupying lesion in the liver on type-B ultrasound and CT during check-up. A tumor 5cm was located in the right posterior lobe of the liver (segment VII) with moderate cirrhosis. A right partial hepatectomy was performed and 5ml anhydrous ethanol injected into the cut surface of the liver by Dr. Zengchen Ma and Dr. Xuecheng Wang in Nov 1993 at age 43. Convalescence was uneventful and AFP decreased from 2,378μg/L to normal. No adjuvant therapy was given. Pathology was HCC. Follow-up by Sep 2015 at age 65, he was in good health with ongoing tumor-free survival of 21 years.

Other Relevant Data

His parents had no hepatitis or liver cancer.

He ranked third among 5 siblings. The eldest brother passed away from liver cancer, the 2nd elder brother and a young brother both died of massive upper gastrointestinal bleeding due to end stage liver cirrhosis. The 5th, his sister is in good health.

He is a very kind-hearted and optimistic person and has a positive attitude on life.

His life is well regulated and liked playing basketball.

He has a wide range of food options and liked pork, seafood, duck eggs, but not chicken, mutton or spicy foods.

His latest check-up on Oct 27 2014, including AFP, chest X-ray, type-B ultrasound and CT were all normal.

Key Points to Remember

His family was the third with many members suffering from liver cancer in this series.

Of the 5 siblings, 2 had liver cancer, 2 had end-stage cirrhosis, and the youngest sister is in good health. Three male siblings had passed away with Mr. Shang still alive after hepatectomy for liver cancer.

It is not very clear, what made a family have many liver cancers. It could be genetic, mother-child transmission, common living conditions, unhealthy foods or polluted water.

His parents had no liver cancer or other liver disease. Carcinogenic factors from the environment should be considered.

With improved living conditions and hepatitis B vaccination, the incidence of liver cancer has shown a downward trend. With advances in medicine, treatment outcome in liver cancer has dramatically improved. Excessive fear of liver cancer is unwarranted.

Up to the present, there is no effective measure to prevent liver cancer. Regular physical check-up including AFP assay and type-B ultrasound of the liver (at least once a year) is helpful in early detection and timely treatment.

Case 74

(Admission No. 273345)
A Single Resection, Ongoing Survival 21 Years
(Feb 1994-   )

Synopsis

Mr. Wang, cadre, was born Nov 1952 in Yiwu, Zhejiang. His AFP was positive during liver cancer survey. Type-B ultrasound and CT showed a space-occupying lesion in the liver. A tumor 4 cm was located in the left lateral lobe of the liver (segment II) with mild cirrhosis. A left lateral segmentectomy was performed by Dr. Zhaoyou Tang and Dr. Fangxian Sun in Feb 1994 at age 41. His AFP decreased from 2,610μg/L to normal.

No adjuvant treatment was given. Pathology was HCC. Follow-up by Sep 2015 at age 62, he was well with ongoing survival of 21 years.

Other Relevant Data

He had HAV hepatitis in 1988, but no family history of liver cancer.

He is optimistic and cheerful. He believed in modern medicine and actively cooperated with his physicians.

He shared his anticancer experiences with other patients without any reserve.

His anticancer story had been reported by the media.

He is retired, but volunteered continue to work.

He is unwilling to be idle and went to the country side to do farm work every weekend in addition to working in the city.

He had a wide range of food options with no special unusual eating habits, smoked and drank occasionally.

Case 75

(Admission No. 275152)
Three Resections, Ongoing Survival 21 Years
(May 1994–   )

Synopsis

Ms. Luo, cadre, was born Jun 1949 in Shanghai. She had 3 resections for liver cancer. When screening for liver cancer she was found to have a space-occupying lesion in the liver on type-B ultrasound and CT. The tumor 4.5cm was located in the right lobe (segments Ⅴ – Ⅵ). A right partial hepatectomy was performed at age 45 by Dr. Zengchen Ma and Dr. Weiqi Lu in May 1994. Chinese Herbal Medicine was given for 1 year and interferon for 1 month. A recurrent tumor 3.5cm in the right lobe was found on type-B ultrasound and CT and a right partial hepatectomy was smoothly performed by Dr. Zengchen Ma and Dr. Huichuan Sun in Oct 1997. In Dec 2012, a small recurrent tumor about 2cm located in the left lateral lobe was detected on contrast enhanced ultrasound and confirmed by MRI. As the tumor was not completely eradicated after 2 interventional treatments, a 3rd operation, a left lateral segmentectomy was performed by Dr. Zengchen Ma and Dr. Qinghai Ye in Apr 2014. Because of extensive adhesions, the operation was quite difficult.

However, convalescence was basically uneventful with a satisfactory outcome. The 3 pathologies were all HCC with nodular cirrhosis. Follow-up by Sep 2015 at age 66, she was well with ongoing survival of 21 years.

Other Relevant Data

This patient had no HBV infection history or family history of liver cancer.

AFP was all negative before resections (8μg/L, 4μg/L and 16μg/L).

All recurrent lesions generally could be detected by type-B ultrasound and confirmed by CT or MRI. At times, contrast enhanced ultrasound is needed to help make the diagnosis.

She lived a regulated life with optimism. Her day began at 6 AM, practiced Tai Chi in the morning, took a nap and cared for her grand-daughter in the afternoon, then went to bed at 10 PM.

She liked to travel and often spent her leisure time with her husband in the beautiful water towns of southern China.

She was very careful with her diet. She did not eat mutton and crabs. She felt the ocean was polluted and did not eat seafood.

Her husband summed up her successful experiences in the treatment of liver cancer as: ① a good team of physicians in a well-equipped hospital, ② a good character and optimism on the part of the patient, cooperating well with her physicians, ③ a supportive harmonious family with each member willing to share all difficulties and ④ a good financial basis to make expenses affordable.

Key Points to Remember

There are 3 outcomes after resection of liver cancer: ① "one resection once for all" with no recurrence or metastasis, ② recurrence and ③ extrahepatic metastasis.

Recurrence and metastasis are expected events in the natural development of liver cancer, no matter how early the disease and how radical the resection. However, the time of their occurrence could not be predicted. Their detection is intimately linked to the quality of follow-up. Once detected, a "never give up" attitude should be adopted and timely appropriate treatment instituted unless contraindicated. This is the only way to realize long-term survival.

Recurrence or metastasis could be detected early only by regular check-up. The protocol consists of AFP monitoring, B-ultrasound, CT or MRI and a chest film. At times, contrast enhanced ultrasound or hepatic arteriography is implemented.

Surgical resection is the most effective mode for treatment of recurrence. When surgery is contraindicated, other modalities should be considered.

This patient has a long-term survival of 21 years after 3 resections indicated strongly recurrence of liver cancer should be treated with a positive aggressive attitude.

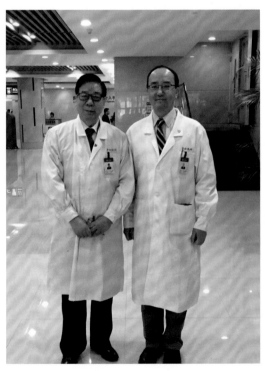

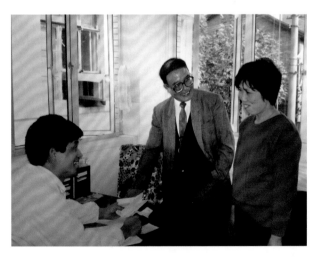

Fig. 1.48   Patient (right) 21 years ongoing survival after 3 liver resections and husband at the Outpatient Clinic 5 months after the 1st resection (Oct 1994)

Fig. 1.49   Surgeons, Dr. Zengchen Ma (left) and Dr. Huichuan Sun　(Feb 2019, Zhongshan Hospital)

Case 76

(Admission No. 276010)
A Single Resection, Ongoing Survival 21 Years
(Jun 1994–   )

Synopsis

Ms. Wu worked in Shanghai. She sought medical care for right upper abdominal discomfort, and a space-occupying lesion in the liver on type-B ultrasound and CT with normal AFP (6μg/L). The tumor 5cm was located in the right anterior lobe of the liver, close to the gallbladder with no cirrhosis. A right partial hepatectomy and cholecystectomy were performed at age 40 by Dr. Zengchen Ma and Dr. Weiqi Lu in Jun 1994. Pathology was poorly differentiated HCC. Follow-up by Sep 2015 at age 61, she was well with ongoing survival of 21 years.

Other Relevant Data

This patient had no HBV infection history. Her parents had no hepatic disease background, but her elder brother died of end stage cirrhosis.

Key Points to Remember

Pathologically, according to Edmondson's classification, hepatocellular carcinoma can be classified into four grades: Grade I highly differentiated; Grade II moderately differentiated; Grade III lowly differentiated and Grade IV undifferentiated. Clinically, Grade II and III HCC are the most common, while Grades I and IV HCC are infrequent. Edmondson's classification criteria are mainly based on cell morphology, nuclear abnormity, bile secretion and tissue structure.Theoretically, the degree of differentiation in HCC affects prognosis. Grade I has the best outcome and Grade IV the worst. In real life, this is not absolute, many other factors also affect prognosis.

Case 77

(Admission No. 277558)
A Single Resection, Ongoing Survival 21 Years
(Aug 1994-   )

Synopsis

Ms. Jin was born Apr 1954 in Nanhui, Shanghai. She sought medical care for upper abdominal discomfort. Her AFP was elevated and type-B ultrasound and CT showed a space-occupying lesion in the liver. The tumor 3cm was located in the left lateral lobe (segment Ⅲ) with no liver cirrhosis. An extended left lateral segmentectomy was carried out by Dr. Zengchen Ma and Dr. Yi Tang in Aug 1994 at age 40. Pathology was poorly differentiated HCC. Traditional Chinese Medicine was given for 10 years. Follow-up by Sep 2015 at age 61, she was in good health with ongoing survival of 21 years.

Other Relevant Data

She had no HBV infection history.

Her AFP decreased from 106μg/L to normal after resection.

In addition to hepatectomy, she underwent 2 other operations, radical resection for rectal cancer in Apr 1993 and total hysterectomy with bilateral salpingo-oophorectomy for leiomyoma of the uterus in Apr 1995. Convalescence was uneventful with satisfactory outcomes.

Her husband died of liver cancer in 1991.

Her daughter is in good health and the mother of a little girl.

Key Points to Remember

This is another long-term survivor after hepatectomy for poorly differentiated HCC. She was treated with Chinese Herbal Medicine post-op. This again sustained our feeling that post-op systemic chemotherapy is not needed even in patients with poorly differentiated HCC.

According to our data, it is very rare for both husband and wife to have liver cancer. This patient's instance was merely a coincidence. Liver cancer is not contagious and isolation is not necessary.

Case 78

(Admission No. 278036)
A Single Resection, Ongoing Survival 21 Years
(Aug 1994⁻　)

Synopsis

Ms. Jiang, fisherwoman, was born Dec 1962 in Wenling, Zhejiang. She was asymptomatic, but AFP-positive on physical check-up. Type-B ultrasound and CT both showed a space-occupying lesion in the liver. The tumor 3.5cm was located in the right lobe (segments V – VIII) and a right partial hepatectomy was performed at age 32 by Dr. Zengchen Ma and Dr. Yi Tang in Aug 1994. Chinese Herbal Medicine was given for 2 years and interferon for 6 months. Pathology was moderately differentiated HCC with no cirrhosis. Follow-up by Sep 2015 at 52, she was in good health with ongoing survival of 21 years.

Other Relevant Data

She had HBV hepatitis and a family history of liver cancer. Her mother and one young brother died of liver cancer in 1995 (age 51) and 1992 (age 27), respectively.

Her AFP returned from 154μg/L to normal after resection.

She is optimistic and cheerful. She believed in modern medicine and actively cooperated with her physicians.

She had a wide range of food options (including chicken and red meat) with no restrictions.

She was born and brought up in a seaside city and had a natural predilection for seafood.

Her husband is a fisherman and in good health. Her son was 10 years old when she had her surgery. He is now married and has a lovely boy (born in 2013). She has become a grandmother and leads a happy life.

Key Points to Remember

This is a family with more than 2 inmates suffering from liver cancer. Onset of liver cancer was irregular among members in the family. The incidence was higher than in a normal family. We feel annual physical check-ups are needed for all members of such a family.

Case 79

(Admission No. 279279)
Two Resections, Ongoing Survival 21 Years
(Oct 1994–   )

Synopsis

Mr. Pan, farmer, was born Mar 1943 in Tongling, Anhui. He sought medical care for right upper abdomen discomfort of 9 months after cholecystectomy. Type-B ultrasound and CT showed a space-occupying lesion in the liver. The tumor 3cm was located in the right posterior lobe (segment Ⅵ) and a right partial hepatectomy was performed at age 51 by Dr. Zengchen Ma and Dr. Qinghai Ye in Oct 1994. Fifteen years later, a palpable upper abdomen mass was diagnosed as recurrent liver cancer, confirmed by type-B ultrasound and CT. The tumor 4.5cm was located in the left lateral lobe. A left hemihepatectomy was carried out by Dr. Zengchen Ma and Dr. Qinghai Ye in Jun 2009 at age 66. Convalescence was basically uneventful with outcome satisfactory. No adjuvant therapy was given after the resections. Pathologies were moderately differentiated HCC with cirrhosis. Follow-up by Sep 2015 at age 72, he was in good health with ongoing survival of 21 years.

Other Relevant Data

He had no hepatitis history and his parents had no liver cancer, but his uncle died of liver cancer.

His AFP was mildly elevated and returned from 32μg/L to normal after the first resection, but was normal (only 1.9μg/L) before the 2nd resection.

Key Points to Remember

This case again proved the importance of follow-up and the value of repeated resection to prolong survival.

Case 80

(Admission No. 280466)
A Single Resection, Ongoing Survival 20 Years
(Nov 1994-   )

Synopsis

Ms. Ling, teacher, was born Jun 1954 in Shanghai. She sought medical care for discomfort in the liver area. AFP was positive and type-B ultrasound as well as CT showed a space-occupying lesion in the liver.

Two separate tumors, each 1.2cm, were located in the right lobe of the liver (segment Ⅷ) and a right partial hepatectomy was performed at age 40 by Dr. Zengchen Ma and Dr. Yumin Zhou in Nov 1994. Convalescence was smooth. Pathology was HCC with mild nodular cirrhosis.

Follow-up by Sep 2015 at 61, she was well with ongoing survival of 21 years.

Other Relevant Data

She was AFP positive and AFP decreased from 750μg/L to normal.

She has a peaceful mentality and is optimistic. She lived a regulated life without unhealthy habits. She has a wide range of food options and preferred seafood with no restrictions. Her favorite hobby is singing. Her husband is a piano teacher. They also often gave music lessons in the community.

Case 81

(Admission No. 280742)
Two Resections, Ongoing Survival 20 Years
(Dec 1994–   )

Synopsis

Mr. Wu, retired naval officer, was born Apr 1956 in Fuding, Fujian. He was referred to a Military Hospital in Fuzhou for a space-occupying lesion in the liver on type-B ultrasound during physical check-up. Primary liver cancer was suspected and he was transferred to Shanghai. Anhydrous ethanol injection was given for the suspected liver cancer at the Second Military Medical University Affiliated Shanghai Oriental Hepato-biliary Surgery Hospital. In Dec 1994 he was admitted to the Shanghai Zhongshan Hospital for operation. The tumor 3.7cm was located in the right lobe of the liver close to the 2nd hepatic hilum. It was 2cm from the IVC and buried 3cm deep in the liver, normally considered a very difficult surgical case. A right partial hepatectomy was performed uneventfully with the aid of intermittent Pringle maneuver by Dr. Zhaoyou Tang and Dr. Zengchen Ma. Convalescence was smooth. Pathology was Grade II differentiated HCC. Interferon was given for 6 months. He was again admitted to the Military Hospital in Fuzhou because of recurrence detected on type-B ultrasound and MRI. He was explored jointly by surgeons from Shanghai Zhongshan Hospital and the local hospital in Dec 2007. The tumor 1.8cm was located in the left medial lobe of the liver. A partial hepatectomy was carried out by Dr. Zengchen Ma and Dr. Yi Jiang. Pathology was HCC. One hundred doses of Cinobufotalin were given orally after the 2nd resection. Follow-up by Sep 2015 at age 59, he was in good health with ongoing survival of 20 years.

Other Relevant Data

This patient had no HBV infection history or family history of liver cancer.

He was AFP negative ($2\mu g/L$) before the 1st resection, but became positive when the tumor recurred. AFP dropped from $105\mu g/L$ to normal after the 2nd resection.

He is cheerful and has a peaceful mentality.

He has a wide range of food options with no restrictions.

His wife and daughter are in good health. His daughter was 12 when he had the 1st surgery. She is now married and the mother of a little girl. Together they lead a happy life.

Key Points to Remember

This case again proved the fact that the biologic characteristics of liver cancer is not set in stone. AFP-positive HCC could become AFP-negative on recurrence (case 46). Similarly, AFP-negative could also become AFP-positive HCC. His AFP was normal before the 1st resection, but became mildly elevated with recurrence. Acknowledgement of this characteristic is helpful in early detection of recurrence. We would like to emphasize again that regular follow-up with both AFP and imaging should be enforced in patients with liver cancer.

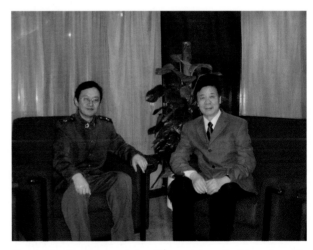

Fig. 1.50   Surgeons of the 2nd resection, Dr. Zengchen Ma (right) and Dr. Yi Jiang (left, Dept. of Surgery, General Military Hospital, Fuzhou) (Dec 2007)

Case 82

(Admission No. 281732)
A Single Resection, Ongoing Survival 20 Years
(Dec 1994–)

Synopsis

Mr. Zheng was born Apr 1951 in Shanghai. He sought medical care for a space-occupying lesion in the liver on type-B ultrasound during physical check-up. He was AFP positive (782μg/L). The tumor 6cm was located in the right lobe (segment Ⅶ) with no cirrhosis. A right partial hepatectomy was performed at age 43 by Dr. Zengchen Ma and Dr. Yumin Zhou in Dec 1994. Pathology was HCC. AFP returned to normal. TCM was given for 7 years. Follow-up by Sep 2015 at age 64, he was in good health with ongoing survival of 20 years.

Other Relevant Data

This patient had both HBV hepatitis and family history of liver cancer.

He was born and grew up in a family with high liver cancer incidence. Two uncles, an elder brother and a young sister all died of liver cancer. An elder sister (case 42 in our series) is still alive with ongoing survival of 28 years after hepatectomy and adjunctive treatment. Another young sister in the USA is in good health with ongoing tumor-free survival of 15 years after liver transplantation for liver cancer and end stage cirrhosis.

He is optimistic and cheerful. He believed in modern medicine and actively cooperated with his physicians.

He has a wide range of food options with no restrictions.

He often helped others and received compliments from relatives and friends. In 2008, he was invited to Germany for a 3-month tour by his father-in-law.

His wife and son are in good health. His son born in 1986, is now married and father of a lovely boy (in 2013).

Key Points to Remember

Salvage of the patient and his two sisters with liver cancer is due to development of liver surgery and liver transplantation.

Surgical treatment is still the most important approach for liver cancer until the advent of new effective medical treatment in the future.

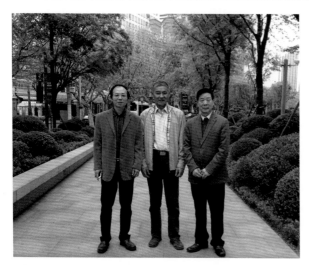

Fig. 1.51   Twenty years ongoing survival after a single resection. 20th post-op year (Apr 2015) Patient (middle）and surgeons, Dr. Ma (right) and Dr. Ye (left)

Case 83

(Admission No. 281915)
A Single Resection, Ongoing Survival 20 Years
(Dec 1994−   )

Synopsis

Ms. Xu, warehouse janitor, was born Apr 1953 in Ningbo, Zhejiang and worked in Hangzhou. She sought medical care for a space-occupying lesion in the liver on type-B ultrasound during physical check-up. She was referred to Shanghai Zhongshan Hospital and explored. The tumor 3cm was located in the right lobe (segment Ⅴ) beside the gallbladder. A right partial hepatectomy with cholecystectomy was performed at age 41 by Dr. Zengchen Ma and Dr. Qinghai Ye in Dec 1994. TCM was given for 6 years. Pathology was HCC. Annual check-up (AFP, B-ultrasound and chest X-ray) was normal. Follow-up by Sep 2015 at age 61, she was well with ongoing survival of 20 years.

Other Relevant Data

This patient had no HBV infection history or family history of liver cancer.

She was AFP negative.

She is optimistic, cheerful and unscheming.

She had no specific eating habits or restrictions. She liked meat, especially pork.

She was a blessed person, turned misfortune into good luck. The whole family cared for her. Her daughter took care of her grandson, and her husband did all the housework. She liked to surf the internet, watch Video plays and chat with friends. She especially loved to sing pop songs by the banks of West Lake.

Case 84
(Admission No. 282311)
A Single Resection, Ongoing Survival 20 Years
(Jan 1995-)

Synopsis

Mr. Zhao, cadre, was born May 1948 in Nanchang, Jiangxi. He sought medical care for discomfort in the liver area. Type-B ultrasound and CT showed a space-occupying lesion in the liver. The tumor 9cm was located in the right lobe (segments V – VI) with no cirrhosis. A right partial hepatectomy was performed at age 47 by Dr. Zenghen Ma and Dr. Qinghai Ye in Jan 1995. Pathology was moderately differentiated HCC. TACE was given and TCM administered for 6 years. Follow-up by Sep 2015 at age 67, he was well with ongoing survival of 20 years.

Other Relevant Data

He had acute icteric hepatitis in 1968, but no family history of liver cancer.

He was AFP negative (7μg/L).

He had no specific eating habits or restrictions and did not smoke nor drink. He liked meat, especially pork.

He liked to play table tennis and took part in matches. He won the 2nd place at a match in Nanchang.

He liked to write poetry to express his feelings after overcoming cancer and his gratitude to the medical staff.

His wife and daughter are in good health. His daughter was 9 when he had his surgery. She is now married and the mother of a little boy.

He felt very happy and thought he was handsome with his daughter looked like him and the grandson looked like his daughter. The 3 generations lead a happy life.

Key Points to Remember

TACE was employed as a prophylactic measure post-op because the tumor was rather large and bore a greater risk of recurrence.

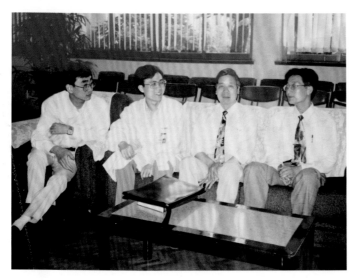

Fig. 1.52 Surgeons of this patient: Dr. Zengchen Ma (2nd, right), Dr. Qionghai Ye (2nd, left), Dr. Xiaowu Huang (1st, right) and Surgical Doctoral graduate student (1st, left) Jun 1996

Case 85

(Admission No. 282783)
Two Resections, Ongoing Survival 20 Years
(Feb 1995–   )

Synopsis

Mr. Xiao, technician, was born Mar 1950 in Shanghai. When screening high-risk liver cancer subjects, he was found to have a space-occupying lesion in the liver on type-B ultrasound. CT confirmed the finding. The tumor 7.5cm was located in the right lobe (segment Ⅶ). A right partial posterior lobectomy was performed at age 45 by Dr. Zengchen Ma and Dr. Guangrong Cai in Feb 1995. He also had an adjuvant TACE. Nine years later, recurrence occurred and was detected on type-B ultrasound. The tumor 2.5cm was located in the right lobe close to the 2nd hepatic hilum. A right partial hepatectomy was performed and 8 ml anhydrous ethanol injected into the cut surface of the liver by Dr. Zengchen Ma and Dr. Qinghai Ye in Sep 2004. He had another TACE and interferon was administered for 3 years. Pathologies were HCC.

Unfortunately, a year later, in Nov 2005 a tumor 2.2 cm again recurred. Because the tumor clung to the IVC with no clear margin, combined alternative treatments were instituted instead of resection. Under ultrasound-guided anhydrous alcohol injections, hepatic artery interventional therapy, gamma-Knife (at a Military Hospital), external radiotherapy, interferon, etc. were administered. Follow-up by Sep 2015 at age 65, he was stable and became a tumor-bearing survivor with ongoing survival of 20 years.

Other Relevant Data

This patient had HBV hepatitis in 1985, but no family history of liver cancer.

He was persistently AFP negative, but elevated from 53μg/L to 135μg/L between Aug 2014 and Aug 2015.

He had no specific eating habits or restrictions.

He liked to share with other patients anticancer experiences without any reserve.

He is a devout and kindhearted Christian.

His favorite hobby is singing and likes to sing traditional Shanghai Opera, at times, to entertain his relatives and friends.

His wife and son are in good health. His son born in 1980, graduated from a prestigious university has a good job and is the father of a lovely boy (in 2012). He leads a happy life in his old age.

Key Points to Remember

Surgical resection is the most effective way to treat liver cancer.

In certain patients, no matter how thorough the resection, recurrence was still unavoidable.

Recurrence could be treated by resection or comprehensive modalities.

Liver transplantation could be a good option for recurrence when all therapies failed or large blood vessels were involved or there was severe cirrhosis.

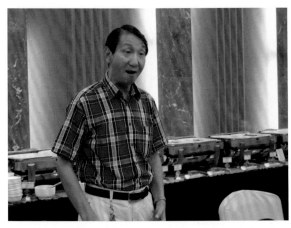

Fig. 1.53   Patient, 20 years ongoing survival after two resections. Patient liked singing and often sang Traditional Shanghai Opera to entertain friends and fellow patients (Aug 2014)

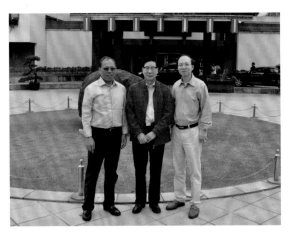

Fig. 1.54   Surgeons: Dr. Zengchen Ma (middle), Dr. Yumin Zhou (left, Surgical Fellow of Shanghai No.1 People's Hospital) and Dr. Qinghai Ye (right), Oct 2015

Case 86

(Admission No. 285127)

A Single Resection, Ongoing Survival 20 Years

（May 1995–　）

Synopsis

Mr. Li, farmer, was born Aug 1936 in Yongkang, Zhejiang. The patient had 3 malignancies, underwent 3 major operations and achieved long-term survival. In May 1988 at age 51, he had resection of rectal cancer at the Jinhua Central Hospital in Zhejiang. In Feb 1990 at age 53, he had radical colectomy for transverse colon cancer at the same hospital. Pathologies were adenocarcinoma. In May 1995 at age 58, he had a hepatectomy for liver cancer at Shanghai Zhongshan Hospital. The tumor 4.5cm was located in the right lobe. A right partial hepatectomy was performed by Dr. Zengchen Ma and Dr. Yingqiang Shi. Pathology was Grade Ⅱ–Ⅲ differentiated HCC. No adjuvant treatment was given. Follow-up by Sep 2015 at age 78, he was well with ongoing survival of 20 years after liver resection.

Other Relevant Data

This patient had no HBV infection history or family history of liver cancer.

He was AFP negative, 2μg/L.

He had no specific eating habits or restrictions.

His wife and 3 sons are in good health.

He continued to do farm work in the fields after the operations.

Key Points to Remember

It is uncommon for a patient to have 2 metachronous colorectal cancers. It is very important to have regular CEA monitoring and colonoscopy after resection of colorectal cancer.

Liver is the most common site of colorectal cancer metastasis.

However, a space-occupying lesion in the liver is not necessarily secondary liver cancer after colorectal cancer resection. This patient supported the above view. His liver lesion was not secondary, but primary.

Regardless of primary or secondary liver cancer, the best treatment is surgery.

The patient suffered in succession 3 malignancies: rectal, colon and liver. His luck was bad. But with surgery and his tenacious perseverance in his struggle with cancer, he finally won and led a long life. This was a very unusual case. It reflected the progress in modern medicine and also the strong will of the patient in his battle against cancer.

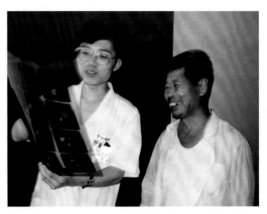

Fig. 1.55   Patient, 20 years ongoing survival after a single resection for liver cancer. Photo: Dr. Qinghai Ye (left) and patient (right) at Outpatient Clinic of Zhongshan Hospital, Aug 1996

Case 87

(Admission No. 286403)
A Single Resection, Ongoing Survival 20 Years
(Sep 1995–   )

Synopsis

Mr. Chen, cadre, was born Dec 1932 in Nahui, Shanghai. He sought medical care for a space-occupying lesion in the liver on type-B ultrasound during physical check-up. CT scanning confirmed the finding and liver cancer was suspected. In Sep 1995 at age 62, operation found the tumor 5cm located in the right lobe (segment V), close to the gallbladder. A right partial hepatectomy and cholecystectomy were performed by Dr. Zengchen Ma and Dr. Qinghai Ye. No adjuvant treatment was given. Pathology was moderately differentiated HCC. Follow-up by Sep 2015 at age 82, he was well with ongoing survival of 20 years.

Other Relevant Data

This patient had HBV hepatitis in 1978, but no family history of liver cancer.

He was AFP negative (2μg/L).

He lived a regulated life. He got up at 6 AM, went to bed at 9 PM and insisted taking a walk every day.

He is a retired cadre, reads newspapers every day and cared about domestic and international events.

He lived with his wife, but not his children and did not need their care.

He is optimistic, cheerful and has a peaceful mentality.

His way of keeping good health was self massage. The sites were nose, ear, chest, abdomen and perineum.

He was willing to share his anticancer experiences with other patients without any reserve.

He had no specific eating habits or restrictions, but has a sweet tooth.

His elder son's daughter made her grandfather a great-grandfather in Jan. 2015. He is a venerable old man and the 4 generations live a happy life.

He felt very happy, rejoiced in the cure of liver cancer to begin a new life. His wish was to invite the medical staff that took care of him to his hometown for vacation to breathe the fresh air, enjoy the local scenery and taste delicious fruits.

Case 88

(Admission No. 287805)
Two-Step Resection of Liver Lymphoma, Ongoing Survival 20 Years
(Jul 1995–   )

Synopsis

Mr. Jiang, was born 1982 in Zhejiang. He was referred to Shanghai due to space-occupying lesions in the liver on type-B ultrasound and CT. He was suspected to have liver cancer and was explored jointly by surgeons from the Zhongshan Hospital and SMU Affiliated Children's Hospital in Jul 1995 at age 12. Tumors were multiple, unequal in size and distributed throughout the liver with enlarged hilar lymph nodes. A palliative procedure, cannulation of the variant right hepatic artery and ligation of the variant right hepatic and common hepatic arteries with needle biopsy was performed by Dr. Zengchen Ma. Pathology was malignant lymphoma. Chemotherapy via the variant right hepatic artery was given. A month later, chemotherapy was discontinued due to blockage of the catheter. Subsequently, 5 courses of CTX, ADM, VCR, PRED systemic chemotherapy were administered. A year later. Surprisingly, imaging found there was only a single tumor left and all others disappeared. During 5 years of follow-up, the disease was stable, but the lone tumor remained unchanged. A 2nd operation was carried out in Mar 2000 at age 17. The tumor 1.6 cm was located in the right lobe with no cirrhosis or enlarged hilar lymph nodes. A right partial hepatectomy was performed by Dr. Zhiquan Wu and the hepatic artery catheter removed. Pathology was coagulation necrosis. The procedure was basically smooth, except for a wound infection that healed uneventfully. Surprisingly, In Jun 2006, 6 years after the 2nd operation, the healed incision full-thickness dehisced spontaneously. It was repaired under intravenous anesthesia and healed quickly.

Follow-up by Sep 2015 at age 32, he was alive with ongoing survival of 20 years.

Other Relevant Data

He is now an entrepreneur and his business being challenged by online shopping.

He is very busy and leads an irregular life, often goes to bed late.

He had no specific eating habits or restrictions and still smoked and drank wine.

He has 3 healthy, smart and pretty children.

His parents and wife are in good health and the 3 generations live a happy life.

Key Points to Remember

The right hepatic artery anomaly in this case did cause some concern at the beginning. Because the normally located right hepatic artery was very slim and stenosed, we had to look for its variant. The mutated right hepatic artery was rather large, arose from the superior mesenteric artery and coursed behind the hepatoduodenal ligament.

This was a case of very successful treatment of malignant lymphoma.

Malignant lymphoma of the liver is very rare and is often multiple. It is not necessarily accompanied by extrahepatic lymphoma.

Malignant lymphoma of the liver is also sensitive to systemic chemotherapy. We feel hepatic artery ligation and intra-arterial chemotherapy could enhance the efficacy of chemotherapy with less adverse effects. It also should be noted that primary and secondary liver cancer could not be cured with only systemic chemotherapy.

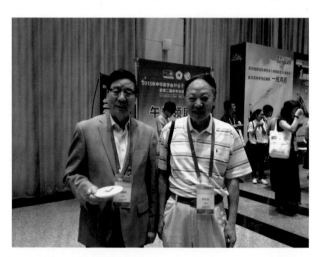

Fig. 1.56   Surgeons involved in 20 years ongoing survival of malignant liver lymphoma, Dr. Zengchen Ma (left, 1st operation, July 1995) And Dr. Zhiquan Wu (right, 2nd operation, Mar 2000) at a surgical conference in Shanghai Jun 2016

Part II

Profile of 88 Cases with Long-Term Survival

All 88 cases were operated between 1961–1995 at Shanghai Zhongshan Hospital and diagnosis confirmed by pathology. Up to Sep 2015, they have survived for 20 or more years. The vast majority of patients were followed or operated on by the authors. Those without complete data and follow-up less than 20 years were not included.

Among them, 85 cases were primary liver cancer, 1 hepatic malignant lymphoma and 2 secondary liver cancer from colon cancer. There were 64 males. The median age was 47 years (1.5–70 years). There were 52 cases (59.1%, 52/88) of small liver cancer (less than 5cm in diameter). The smallest was 1.4cm. Six cases were huge liver cancer (10–15cm) and 7 cases giant liver cancer (more than 15cm). Five cases had cancer thrombi and another 5 pulmonary metastases. Sixty-three (79.7%, 63/79) were AFP-positive. The lowest level of AFP positive was 26μg/L with the highest 80,000μg/L. Sixteen had a family history of liver cancer (18.8%, 16/85). Only a single resection was performed in 63 cases, 2 resections in 13 cases and 3 resections in 2 cases. The two-step operation for large liver cancer was performed in 8 cases. Hepatic artery ligation and cannulation only was performed in 2 cases. Liver resection and resection of subsequent pulmonary metastasis were performed in 5 cases.

In total, there were 117 operations (including pulmonary resections) in the 88 cases. Eight survived 40 or more years with the longest 48 years. Sixteen survived 30–40 years. Sixty-two cases are still alive. Four aged 90 or more years but only 2 still alive. The oldest lived to 99 years at the last follow-up and still living and well.

Part III

Gems to Take Home Experiences and Therapeutic Approaches

It is very difficult to provide accurate figures of long-term survival in liver cancer. The definitive final outcome of each patient should be known. Data collection is hampered by many uncontrollable conditions. To mention a few, data can only be obtained through unrelenting follow-up of patients. The utmost importance of follow-up is sometimes not fully acknowledged by both physician and patient. Consequently, nonadherence is common. In addition, changes in society especially city planning with the accompanied upheaval and turmoil often brought about displacement, migration, relocation and resettlement of the population. A patient is often lost to follow-up, especially when the physician-patient communication bond had not been firmly established.

Furthermore, liver cancer is a costly disease. Its treatment involves a large sum of money. China is still a developing country, most people are not affluent and the scope of coverage by medical insurance is limited. Many patients dropped out halfway through due to financial reasons.

However, the 88 cases reported here can be considered data complete, as they are the personal experiences of the authors, who even traveled long distances to acquire the necessary data. The work was tedious and tiring but rewarding. Actually, these cumulative data could be considered a reflection of the evolution of present day state-of-art in surgical hepatic oncology at Shanghai Zhongshan Hospital.

Among the authors own patients including those with incomplete data that survived for 20 or more years accounted for about 10%.

What is high quality treatment in liver cancer? We feel it should be reflected in the increasing number of long-term survivors and in improvement of patient's quality of life. In a word, it can only be reflected in the liver cancer patient. However, unfortunately this view is not widely shared.

In this study, our goal is to summarize the successful experiences in liver cancer treatment through the large number of cases seen at Shanghai Zhongshan Hospital. Tit for tat, the proverb "use a stone to trade for a gem" prompted us to share our meager successful experiences hoping fellow investigators could also share theirs to enrich our knowledge of liver cancer.

Forty years ago, liver cancer was considered deadly and incurable with liver cancer surgery still unborn. However, through the years, we not only obtained great achievements in liver surgery, but also have had breakthroughs in the therapeutic concept of liver cancer. We firmly believe through the sharing of such experiences, we can further improve our treatment results to the benefit of the patient.

3.1   Hepatectomy is the Most Important Treatment for Liver Cancer. Long-Term Survival is Possible after a Single Resection

All 88 cases underwent surgical treatment and 86 received resection. Sixty-three had only a single resection. Among these 63, 61 were primary liver cancer and 2 secondary liver cancer. The majority of them (61/63) had a single lesion with 2 lesions in only 2 cases. The largest tumor was 17 cm and 4 cases had concomitant tumor thrombi. They were all long-term survivors with only a few with residual tumor.

Early scholars advocated the classic resection for liver cancer, i.e. regular hepatectomy or anatomic hepatectomy, including left lateral lobectomy, left hemi-hepatectomy, right hemi-hepatectomy and right trisectionectomy. To avoid unnecessary major resection, hepatic segmentectomy is suggested to cure small tumors, including single segmentectomy and multi- segmentectomies. The latter procedures also belong to the category of regular hepatectomy.

The newest development in liver cancer surgery is irregular hepatectomy which has become presently the mainstay procedure.

Among the 61 cases with a single lesion, 40 were in the right liver, 20 in the left liver, and 1 in the middle lobe. Irregular hepatectomy was 93% (37/40) of procedures performed for cancer in the right liver. In total, irregular hepatectomy accounted for 69% (42/61) of all hepatic resections.

With accumulation of experience, at times, cancer adjacent to major vessels and when growth expansion caused displacement, distortion and partial compression–occlusion of the latter are still all surgical indications. Of the 117 procedures, 13 were highly difficult, but they all yielded good results.

Because of breakthrough in the concept of liver cancer resection and advances in technology, surgical indications have become less rigid and safety of operation improved.

It is gratifying long-term survivors of more than 20 years reached the goal of "a resection once for all". A single resection accounted for 72% (63/88) of cases.

Although there are many new treatment options for HCC, such as radiofrequency ablation, microwave coagulation and various other methods and medications, the key role of surgical resection in improving long-term outcomes cannot be replaced.

Our conclusion is hepatectomy for liver cancer plays a key role in improving the long-term survival rate of liver cancer. However, the success of treatment requires expertise and a brand new concept of liver cancer surgery.

3.2 Follow-Up Treatment with Resection of Recurrence Can Further Improve Therapeutic Efficacy

We feel recurrence after resection is mainly determined by the biologic characteristics of liver cancer. Of course, rough surgical technique as well as excessive handling of tumor during surgery are also more likely to have recurrence. We would once again like to emphasize that regular follow-up should be maintained after surgery, to detect early recurrence and timely undertake appropriate treatment, especially resection.

Pioneer clinicians long ago recognized the necessity and value of repeated resection for recurrence. Outcomes have greatly improved, survival extended and even obtained a "two-resection once for all", curative effect.

Ten cases in this group survived for 20 or more years after a second resection. The longest survival was 44 years (case 3, but died of bladder cancer). Case 9 is still alive and well after the second resection with a long-term survival of 40 years.

Postoperative follow-up is performed with ultrasound, CT or MRI. The advantages of ultrasound are convenient, economic, time-saving and non-invasive as well as result immediately available. Accurate diagnosis by B-ultrasound depends on the experience and expertise of the performer. However, blind zones and lack of fine detail do exist in ultrasound imaging. To remedy such deficiencies, CT or MRI should be supplemented, especially in B-ultrasound negative instances to avoid a missed diagnosis and when to define 3D anatomic spatial relations in detail is required. AFP assay is another MUST item, irrespective of preoperative AFP being positive or negative. The biologic characteristics could change when a tumor recurs. In other words, AFP negative liver cancer could become AFP-positive, and vice versa.

We feel a patient after the second resection for recurrence should continue be closely followed-up, to detect further recurrence and institute another resection if necessary.

From these 88 cases, we feel one can at least preliminarily surmise there is no apparent correlation between tumor size, AFP level, episodes of recurrence, distant metastasis and prognosis. Furthermore, good outcome and long-term survival can only be realized through surgery and persistent unrelenting lifelong follow-up of the patient with timely management of any detrimental condition when it appears.

Before any operation for recurrence, we should evaluate the risk and prognosis of the procedure, i.e. determine whether the operation is worth while. If the tumor is multiple, too large, or with cancer thrombi and the patient too old and frail, then the resection should not be undertaken. Under the above circumstances, treatment should only be supportive and to alleviate suffering. Unwarranted surgery and aggressive intervention not only would increase suffering and even hasten the patient's demise.

3.3 Long-Term Survival after 3 Successive Hepatectomies for Liver Cancer Further Strengthened the Value of Follow-up Treatment

The third hepatectomy is an active follow-up treatment for the 2nd recurrence. People often simply theorized that the 3rd liver cancer resection would be almost worthless. In fact, effect of the 3rd operation has proved to be very optimistic. For example, case 75, Ms. Luo underwent 3 surgeries, the 1st in 1994, the 2nd 1997, and the 3rd 2014. Follow-up by Sep 2015, she ongoing survived 21 years. In addition, 2 other cases (not in this series) also left a deep impression on us. Both Mr. Li and Mr. Liu underwent a third hepatectomy 14 years (Mar 2001) and 8 years ago (Sep 2007) respectively. Follow-up by Sep 2015, they were all alive and well with an ongoing survival of 19 and 16 years.

Case 22 is similar. Patient underwent the 3rd operation for recurrence 6 years (1986) after a two-step resection. The operation once again extended his life with an ongoing survival of 35 years. All these sufficiently demonstrated the important value of the 3rd operation. We feel that for patients with recurrence, including those after a two-step resection, follow-up should not be given-up and neglect the 3rd surgical treatment. Of course, we should avoid a blind 3rd operation when there is no strong indication.

Technically, a 3rd resection is more difficult than the 2nd and requires higher overall judgment, higher surgical skills and more meticulous post-op care.

We can select other options for the 2nd recurrence, but resection is the most important and beneficial. To date, there is no ideal way to prevent recurrence. Therefore, we emphasize here again, the importance of postoperative follow-up. Without a sound concept of follow–up, there is no other way to obtain good results and long-term survival.

3.4   Long-Term Survival after Liver Cancer Resection and Resection of Pulmonary Metastasis Again Highlighted the Value of Follow-up with Definitive Treatment

Lung is the most frequently involved organ in liver cancer. Metastasis to the lung after liver resection is not uncommon. Two different opinions exist regarding the surgical treatment of lung metastasis. One is relatively negative. It is believed that lung metastasis is a late manifestation of cancer and surgical treatment of no benefit. Whereas the other view is positive. Surgical treatment for lung metastasis is valuable.

We feel it is necessary to take a positive attitude towards isolated and localized pulmonary metastasis and treat it in time, especially by surgical resection.

In our 88 cases, we performed pulmonary resection for metastases in cases 8, 10, 12 and 28 as well as mediastinal resection in addition for metastasis after a two-step resection in case 42. Their lives were extended by 28, 22, 35, 19 and 21 years, respectively. Their total survivals were 32, 25, 40, 20 and 28 years, respectively. The above suggested that treatment of lung metastasis in a liver cancer patient, especially by resection has important value in achieving long-term survival.

With advances in technology and the advent of the thoracoscope, a small metastatic lesion can be removed by mini invasive thoracoscopy with good results.

In addition to lung, adrenal gland is also a frequent metastatic site. Treatment principle is the same, remove it promptly and thoroughly.

It must be emphasized a chest film should be taken every 6 months post-op, in addition to the regular ultrasound imaging, CT scan and AFP assay. From our data, most lung metastasis occurred within 5 years after the liver resection. However, we feel that, even after 5 years, chest films should still be taken regularly.

We have gained 2 major understandings in the aggressive resection of lung metastasis in liver cancer. First, resection can cure patients with lung metastasis. Second, in depth scientific understanding of the nature of lung metastasis: ① lung metastasis can exist alone, not necessarily co-exist with a recurrence in the liver; ② lung metastasis can be solitary, not necessarily multiple; and ③ lung metastasis does not mean there is already spread to the whole body. For example case 12, after pulmonary resection, "one resection for all", the survival was extended by 35 years (total ongoing survival 40 years). If confounded by groundless irrational thinking and no action is taken, the patient could not have lived happily for such a long time.

However, there is a limit to the "Never Give Up". Risks should never exceed benefit and the latter is always the priority when assessing a patient. We should have a "limit" concept in surgical resection in such patients. Unlimited extension of surgical indication, neglecting risk and benefit, unwarrantly carry out palliative resection of metastatic lesions would not only be unhelpful but also harmful.

It should be emphasized that resection of lung metastasis is not always "one resection for all". There is still a possibility of recurrence. It would be best to continue active follow-up these patients for life.

Mr. Pan's (case 28) treatment experience supported the above view. The patient underwent resection of liver cancer in 1984 and left pulmonary resection for metastasis in 1985. After 6 years, cancer again recurred and a left lateral hepatectomy was carried out (1991). Because the patient underwent 3 surgeries, his life was prolonged from 1 to 7, and then to 20 years. Unfortunately, at age 80, he died of senility but not liver cancer.

Case 42 is similar. Ms. Zheng, in Oct 1986 underwent hepatic artery ligation with cannulation followed by infusion chemotherapy for two big liver cancers. In Feb 1988 the tumors significantly shrank and a two-step resection was carried out. In 1994 pulmonary metastasis and mediastinal metastasis were detected and resected. Since then, she survived for 20 years. However, the tumor recurred again in 2014.

The tumors in the left lobe and right anterior lobe were treated with radiofrequency ablation. Follow-up by Sep 2015, her AFP was normal with tumors completely necrotic on ultrasound and MRI. Her ongoing survival was 28 years.

3.5 Long-Term Survival by Two-Step Liver Resection after Hepatic Artery Ligation with Cannulation and Intra-Arterial Infusion Chemotherapy to "Modify" the Cancer

Although hepatic artery ligation and intra-arterial chemotherapy are not universally accepted and widely used, we feel that this therapeutic modality is very valuable and is one of the revived developments in Surgical Hepatic Oncology. In our data, 8 patients underwent the 2-step resection. They are cases 22, 38, 42, 43, 51, 55, 57 and 88 with survival of 35, 29, 28, 28, 27, 26, 24 and 20 years respectively. Seven of them were primary liver cancer with the remaining (case 88) malignant lymphoma of the liver. Follow-up by Sep 2015, they were all alive. If they underwent a single stage resection or nonoperative treatment, outcome would not have been so good with long-term survival.

Miraculously, 2 other cases (case 24 and case 35) underwent only hepatic artery surgery without resection also obtained long-term survivals of 32 and 25 years respectively. The advantages of hepatic artery surgery compared with other therapies are: possibly induced alteration in characteristics of the cancer, tumor volume reduced, created conditions for resection and finally achieved long-term survival.

A 2-step resection of liver cancer after hepatic artery ligation with cannulation is a kind of treatment strategy simulating that usually adopted in battle or warfare. It reduces tumor size first and then carries out the resection. The rationale is that due to the cut off of blood supply, the tumor's natural character undergoes changes. Its deleterious effects are weakened and subdued. Ultimately the tumor reduced in size is resected and completely eradicated. How to make the liver cancer shrink and its activity decline? At present, the best way is to block its blood supply by ligation of the hepatic artery. Blood supply of liver cancer comes mainly from the hepatic artery. It has been proven that after blocking the hepatic artery, the tumor grows slowly, stops growing or even shrinks in size. However, the effect of hepatic artery therapy varies from person to person. It depends on the completeness of hepatic artery occlusion and tolerance of the tumor with this treatment. In order to enhance assault on the tumor, postoperative intra-arterial chemotherapy can be added. Overall, hepatic artery ligation with infusion chemotherapy is superior to transcatheter arterial chemoembolization (TACE). There are advantages and disadvantages in both treatments. The disadvantage of hepatic artery surgery is its relative complexity and long course of treatment. Both physicians and patients need to have enough patience and perseverance. The basics in this field will be described in detail in chapters that follow.

3.6　Liver Resection Followed by Local Treatment for Liver Cancer is a New Approach to Prolong Survival

Local treatments of liver cancer usually include radiofrequency ablation (RF), microwave, cryotherapy, ethanol injection, gamma knife stereotactic radiotherapy, etc. Although the efficacy of these treatments is not as good as surgical resection, it is much better than chemotherapy and TACE with much less risk than surgery.

In our data, several cases obtained long-term survival by combination of liver resection and local treatment. Take case 54 for example, she had 2 isolated tumors 8cm and 2.5cm in size, separately located in the right lower part (segment Ⅵ) and right upper part (segment Ⅷ) of the liver close to the second hilum. Right partial hepatectomy for the large tumor and 15ml anhydrous ethanol injection into the small tumor were performed. The patient recovered well with no complications. For 26 years

(1988–2014) she lived a happy life with no recurrence or metastasis. Unfortunately, she died of senile dementia in Jan 2015, at age 82. It can be predicted that the effect would not have been so good without anhydrous ethanol injection for the small liver cancer near the second hilum.

We feel anhydrous alcohol injection is effective and simple. We sometimes inject anhydrous alcohol (about 10ml) into the cut surface after resection to kill possible residual cancer cells. This can also achieve good results. A good curative effect can also be obtained by alcohol injection into a small recurrence

Radiofrequency ablation (RFA) is a local treatment for cancer. Under the guidance of B-ultrasound a RFA needle is percutaneously inserted into the liver tumor. The RFA machine is then started to heat the tumor and lead to necrosis. This treatment is very effective and can achieve curative effects in some cancers. The intra-tumor temperature and heating duration can be regulated according to tumor size. In our Liver Cancer Unit this treatment began in 2001. Initially, it was only part of the comprehensive treatment and as a supporting measure. It is now a primary treatment and can even replace surgical resection in certain patients.

Case 42 was a patient with recurrence after multiple operations for liver cancer. The most recent recurrence was treated by RFA. In Mar 2014, B-ultrasound found two recurrent lesions, one 2.8cm in the right anterior lobe and another 1.4cm in the left medial lobe. These were confirmed by MRI and AFP (100μg/L). RFA was applied to the two lesions in Jun 2014. The procedure was successful and outcome satisfactory. B-ultrasound and MRI found no blood supply to the two lesions, denoting tumor necrosis. AFP reduced to normal. Follow-up by Sep 2015 at age 75, she remained stable, AFP normal with no further recurrence and with ongoing survival of 28 years.

RFA can be used alone or as part of comprehensive treatment, such as together with hepatic artery interventional therapy.

RFA can also be applied with laparotomy to facilitate its application.

Needle insertion can be precise and accurate with risk reduced. With the abdomen open, RFA may be used alone, coupled with liver resection and/or hepatic artery surgery as dictated by the presenting situation.

But this treatment has its limitations and certain risks. A large tumor, multiple tumors or the tumor close to the hepatic hilum are not suitable. Complications such as bleeding and bile leakage should be avoided.

3.7 Long-Term Survival after Hepatectomy with Transcatheter Arterial Chemoembolization for Liver Cancer

Transcatheter arterial chemoembolization (TACE) usually refers to hepatic artery chemoembolization. Since 1978, we have developed hepatic arteriography and TACE for liver cancer. The method is under X-ray monitoring a special sterile catheter is inserted selectively or superselective from the femoral artery into the celiac artery, common or proper hepatic artery. A contrast agent is injected to delineate the tumor and its blood supply. The embolic agents, iodized oil, gelatin sponge and chemical drugs are injected into the blood vessels that supply the tumor.

TACE is far less effective than liver resection or local treatment and often plays only a supporting role. Among the 88 long-term survivors, some patients were treated by resection with TACE. We feel pre-op TACE can improve the resection effect and reduce recurrence. However, if pre-op TACE is unduly overemphasized, at times, the optimal time for resection could be lost. Whether surgical resection must be combined with TACE should be tailored rather than generalized.

Post-op TACE can be prophylactic or therapeutic. Prophylactic TACE is the equivalent of "sweeping the battlefield" and "checking for missed fish". Take case 59 as an example, a 38-year-old male liver cancer patient was explored in Dec 1991. The huge tumor 15cm was in the left lateral lobe with a tumor thrombus in the left hepatic vein and extended into the inferior vena cava. An En Bloc resection of the left lateral lobe, left hepatic vein and tumor thrombus was performed. The operation was difficult, but convalescence uneventful. As the tumor was huge and coupled with a thrombus, he received 3 post-op TACE and TCM therapy. Follow-up by Sep 2015, at age 61, he remained healthy with ongoing survival of 23 years.

Therapeutic TACE is a follow-up treatment for patients after inadequate or suspected inadequate resection. In addition, TACE can control growth of the tumor and prolong the life of patients with recurrent HCC not suitable for resection. Generally, TACE can be performed one or more times at intervals of one or several months.

Usually, TACE is not very damaging to the normal liver, but it is of great risk in patients with severe cirrhosis or arteriovenous fistulae. TACE is a palliative treatment and by merely TACE could only prolong a patient's lifespan, but rarely for more than 20 years.

TACE is less effective than liver resection or local therapy, even hepatic artery surgery (ligation and cannulation). It is almost impossible to expect a 2-step resection of liver cancer with reduced tumor volume after TACE. We were able to perform the 2-step resection only in a few patients who showed reduced tumor volume after TACE for large liver cancer.

One of the most impressive case was a 63-year old female, who had a huge liver cancer in the right lobe on B-ultrasound and CT in May 1994. After 4 TACEs, 7 months later, a miracle occurred, the tumor shrank from 13cm to 6cm and AFP dropped from 790μg/L to 130μg/L. A partial liver resection was performed in Dec 1994. The tumor was hard with 90% necrosis. The procedure was smooth and recovery satisfactory. AFP dropped from 130 to normal. Unfortunately, at age 80 years, in Jun 2011 she died of cerebral infarction with survival of 16 years after liver resection.

Effect of TACE depends not only on expertise and experience, arrangement of the tumor's blood supply is also of importance. When the tumor is supplied by a variety of channels the TACE effect is limited. In order to improve the therapeutic effect of TACE, the latest development is ultra-selective embolization with an ultra-thin catheter. Generally, to achieve good results, by merely TACE therapy is not sufficient. TACE needs to be coupled with other forms of local treatment.

When specific conditions exist, liver transplantation might be indicated to achieve long-term survival in liver cancer

Liver transplantation refers to replacement of a diseased liver with a healthy liver or part of it from another person. Liver transplantation can be divided into live donor liver transplantation (LDLT) and brain death donor liver transplantation (BDDLT) according to donor source. Usually, 2 surgical procedures, classic approach or piggyback technique is implemented. The most commonly used technique is classic orthotopic liver transplantation, in which the diseased liver is removed and replaced with a healthy liver or part of it in the same anatomic location. The supra-hepatic inferior vena cava, infra-hepatic inferior vena cava, portal vein, hepatic artery and common bile duct are reconstructed in sequence.

Mar 1 1963, the 37-year old American surgeon Thomas E. Starzl at the University of Colorado, performed the world's 1st human liver transplantation. He is also known as "the Father of liver transplantation." Liver transplantation was first performed at Ruijing Hospital in China in 1977. At Zhongshan Hospital, the first liver transplantation for liver cancer was performed in 1978, but the patient survived only 33 days. After that, liver transplantation in China was in a state of standstill. With progress of transplantation medicine in the world, liver transplantation revived again and obtained fruitful results since 2001 at Zhongshan Hospital.

Liver transplantation is the only treatment for liver cancer with severe cirrhosis. Transplantation could also be performed for certain cancers located in the hepatic hilum not suitable for hepatectomy. Transplantation is a more radical treatment than hepatectomy.

Since Apr 2001, great advances have been made in liver transplantation at Zhongshan Hospital. The first revived liver transplantation patient for liver cancer by Dr. Jia Fan, Dr. Zhi quan Wu and Dr. Jian Zhou has survived for 14 years (surgery in Apr 2001). According to incomplete statistics, at least 70 patients had survived for 10 or more years after transplantation for liver cancer performed between 2001 and 2005 at our hospital. It is certain that in the future, there would be many more liver cancer patients surviving for 20 or more years after liver transplantation.

Liver transplantation can be used not only as the first option for certain patients with liver cancer, but also for recurrence. One example is Mr. Wang, a 44-year-old physician, underwent right partial hepatectomy for liver cancer with cholecystectomy at Zhongshan Hospital in Sep 2002. The cancer recurred after 10 years. As it was close to the hepatic hilum and co-existed with cirrhosis, he underwent liver transplantation by Dr. Jia Fan and Dr. Jian Zhou in Jun 2012. The operation was difficult, but convalescence uneventful. Follow-up by Sep 2015, he remained healthy with ongoing tumor-free survival of 13 years.

However, it should be borne in mind that, when liver cancer can be cured by resection or other treatments, transplantation should not be blindly undertaken. Transplantation is not only unnecessary, it also is a waste of valuable liver resource.

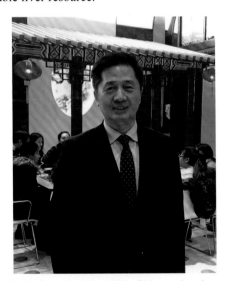

Fig. 3.1   Prof. Jia Fan, Member of the Chinese Academy of Sciences

References

Chen H, Wu MC. 1989. Reoperation of primary liver cancer. In: Tang ZY, Wu MC, Xia SS (eds), Primary liver cancer. Beijing: China Acad Publishers, Berlin: Springer-Verlag, 394-403.

Fan J, Wu ZQ, Tang ZY, et al. 2001. Complete resection of the caudate lobe of the liver with tumor: Technique and experience. Hepato-Gastroenterol, 48: 808-811.

Fan ST, Lo CM, Chan KL, et al. 1996. Liver transplantation-perspective from Hong Kong. Hepato-Gastroenterology, 43: 893-897.

Fortner JG, MacLean BJ, Kim DK, et al. 1981. The seventies evolution in liver surgery for cancer. Cancer, 47(9): 2162-2166.

Foster JH. 1970. Survival after liver resection for cancer. Cancer, 26(3): 493-502.

Friesen SR, Hardin CA, Kittle CF. 1967. Prolonged survivals of ten partial hepatectomies and second look procedures for primary and secondary carcinoma of the liver. Surgery, 61(2): 203-209.

Ikeda K, Saitoh S, Tsubota A, et al. 1993. Risk factors for tumor recurrence and prognosis after curative resection of hepatocellular carcinoma. Cancer, 71: 19-25.

Iwatsuki S, Starzl TE. 1988. Personal experience with 411 hepatic resection. Ann. Surgery, 208(4): 421-434.

Lawrence GH, Grauman D, Lasersohn, et al. 1966. Primary carcinoma of the liver. Amer J Surg, 112(2): 200-210.

Lee NW, Wong J, Ong GB. 1982. The surgical management of primary carcinoma of the liver. World J Surg, 6(1): 66-75.

Lin Chao-ch'i, Yang Yung-chang, et al. 1962. Primary carcinoma of liver, clinical observation on 207 cases. Chinese Medical Journal, 81: 303-314.

Lin TY, Lee CS, Chen KM. 1987. Role of surgery in the treatment of primary carcinoma of the liver. A 31-year experience. Br J Surg, 74(9): 839-842.

Lise M, Bacchetti S, Pian PD, et al. 1998. Prognostic factors affecting long-term outcome after liver resection for hepatocellular carcinoma. Results in a series of 100 Italian patients. Cancer, 82(6): 1028-1036.

Ma ZC, Huang LW, Tang ZY, et al. 2005. "Three-grade criteria" of radical resection for primary liver cancer. Chinese Journal of Clinical Oncology, 2(5): 820-823.

Mazzaferro V, Regalia E, Doci R, et al. 1996. Liver transplantation for the treatment of small hepatocellular carcinomas in patients with cirrhosis. N Engl J Med, 334: 693-699.

Tang ZY, Yu YQ, Zhou XD, et al. 1989. Surgery of small hepatocellular carcinoma.

Analysis of 144 cases. Cancer, 64: 536-541.

Thompson HH, Tompkins RK, Longmire WP. 1983. Major hepatic resection: a 25-year experience. Ann Surg, 197(4): 375-388.

Vauthey JN, Klimstra D, Franceschi D, et al. 1995. Factors affecting long-term outcome after hepatic resection for hepatocellular carcinoma. Am J Surg, 169(1): 28-35.

Wilson E. 1966. Malignant hepatoma: repeated resection of matastases with survival for 15 years. Med J Aust, 2(19): 889-893.

Wu MC, Shen F, Yang JM, et al. 2012. Intergrated treatment of hepatic cancer. In: Gu JR (ed), Primary liver cancer. Hangzhou: Zhejiang University Press, Heidelberg: Springer, 399-431.

Wu ZQ, Fan J, Qiu SJ, et al. 2000. The value of postoperative hepatic regional chemotherapy in prevention of recurrence after radical resection of primary liver cancer. WJG, 6(1): 131-133.

Yu EX, Lu LN. 1989. Traditional Chinese Medicine in liver cancer treatment - Clinical and Experimental Investigation. In: Tang ZY, Wu MC, Xia SS (eds), Primary liver cancer. Beijing: China Acad Publishers, Berlin: Springer-Verlag, 440-448.

Zhou XD, Tang ZY, Ma ZC, et al. 2009. Twenty-year survivors after resection for hepatocellular carcinoma – Analysis of 53 cases. J Cancer Res Clin Oncol, 135: 1067-1072.

蔡光荣, 余业勤, 马曾辰, 汤钊猷, 周信达. 1996. 结直肠肝转移癌手术切除后 11 例远期随访. 中华肿瘤杂志, 18(3): 218-220.

范尚达. 2002. 香港肝脏外科现状. 见：严律南. 肝脏外科. 北京：人民卫生出版社, 1015-1050.

胡宏楷, 吴孟超. 1979. 原发性肝癌术后长期生存 10 年以上的病例分析. 中华肿瘤杂志, 1(1): 47-50.

黄力文, 马曾辰. 2002. 结直肠癌肝转移的外科治疗进展. 中国临床医学, 9(1): 98-100.

黄兴耀, 王能进. 1992. 肝癌术后生存 10 年以上 29 病临床研究. 实用肿瘤杂志, 7(3): 164-166.

李国材. 1988. 从原发性肝癌切除后生存 10 年以上病例试论提高肝癌远期疗效的途径. 癌症, 7(2): 129-131.

林芷英, 汤钊猷, 余业勤, 等. 1991. 原发性肝癌根治性切除术后的复发和治疗. 中华外科杂志, 29(2): 93-96.

刘俊人, 高嘉宏. 2002. 台湾肝细胞癌诊治现状. 见：严律南. 肝脏外科. 北京：人民卫生出版社, 1051-1071.

马曾辰, 汤钊猷, 余业勤, 等. 2001. 原发性肝癌切除后长期生存 113 例报告. 中华普通外科杂志, 16(1): 48-50.

马曾辰. 2003. 肝癌手术与术后长期生存. 中国普外基础与临床杂志, 10(3): 192-193.

马曾辰 吴肇光 汤钊猷. 2008. 肝癌生存 43 年一例. 中华肿瘤杂志, 30(3): 210.

汤钊猷, 余业勤, 周信达, 等. 1992. 1450 例原发性肝癌的外科治疗. 中华外科杂志, 30(6): 325-328.

王成恩, 李国材, 李国辉, 等. 1982. 原发性肝癌外科治疗生存 10 年以上的病例分析 (附 5 例报告). 新医学, 13(8): 396-398.

王学浩, 杜竟辉, 赵中辛, 等. 1997. 肝癌的现代综合治疗 (附 1320 例报告). 中国实用外科杂志, 17(1): 16-18.

严律南, 曾勇, 文天夫, 等. 2000. 1038 例原发性肝癌的外科治疗. 中华外科杂志, 38(7): 520.

Part IV

**Food for Thought on the
Nature of Liver Cancer**

4.1 Liver Cancer is a Systemic Disease as well as Local Disease.

If all malignant tumors were generalized to be systemic diseases, it would greatly discourage people's confidence in conquering cancer. If malignant tumor is not regarded as a systemic disease, blind optimism would greatly affect the final outcome. Therefore, we must vary from person to person, from tumor to tumor and tailor the treatment of cancer

We feel liver cancer in its early stage is mostly a localized disease. Only at a late stage, it would easily spread, metastasize and become systemic. Of the 88 cases, 51 (57.9%) survived for 20 or more years without recurrence after a single liver resection, with the longest ongoing tumor–free survival up to 48 years (case 2).

If liver cancer were a systemic disease, without surgical treatment and by drugs alone, these patients could not have obtained such outcomes.

Accordingly, early recurrence of liver cancer is also considered a local disease, making the 2nd resection rational. In our series, 18 patients (20.5%) with recurrence underwent a 2nd hepatectomy and obtained a "two resections once for all" result. The longest ongoing survival was 40 years.

Based on such understanding, a 3rd surgical resection for recurrence becomes a valid option. In our 88 cases, 4 were cured after the 3rd resection, with the longest ongoing survival of 35 years (case 22).

At the spur of a moment, a hastily made decision without deliberation and based on a misunderstood nature of liver cancer would lead to a completely different therapeutic outcome. Overemphasis on the systemic nature of liver cancer is certainly unfavorable to the patient's benefit.

However, a positive attitude of surgical treatment for early liver cancer does not mean surgery is the only option. Other treatments, such as radiofrequency ablation, microwave therapy, alcohol injection, etc could also be used, depending on the specific situation, such as extent of the disease, condition of the patient, expertise of the physician and facilities available.

One must not mechanically, misunderstand the issue and wrongly consider surgery for patients with multiple foci or advanced liver cancer. This would only not be of benefit, but harmful to the patient. To become a qualified oncologist, one does need to constantly summarize successful experiences and learn lessons from failures to become more competent.

We firmly believe without a devoted dedication on the part of an oncologist, it would hardly be possible to achieve an acceptable quality of life with long-term tumor-free survival in a liver cancer patient.

4. 2　Liver Cancer is a "Ferocious Tiger" as well as a "Big Docile Cat"

Sometimes people like to regard their opponents or enemies as a tiger. What kind of tiger is liver cancer? Without doubt, liver cancer is a real, ferocious tiger. But when we seriously deal with it and beat it, liver cancer is no longer ferocious and terrible. It can be transformed from a ferocious tiger to become a tame big cat.

The successful treatment of 88 cases of liver cancer clearly illustrated the above philosophy.

Mr. Ma (case 59) was a patient with a huge liver cancer and underwent a relatively difficult and complex operation. In Dec 1991 at age 37, the huge tumor 15cm was in the left lobe with a tumor thrombus, 2cm×1cm, in the left hepatic vein and extended into the inferior vena cava. An En Bloc hepatectomy including the left lateral lobe as well as left hepatic vein and thrombus was performed. The operation was difficult, but he recovered well. As the tumor was huge and with a thrombus, he received 3 post-op arterial chemoembolization and TCM therapy. Follow-up by Sep 2015 at age 61, he remained healthy with ongoing tumor-free survival of 23 years.

Mr. Ye was another patient that experienced a very dangerous liver resection (case 66). In Mar 1993 at age 48, exploration found the tumor 6.5cm was located in the right antero-superior lobe (segment Ⅷ) close to the second hepatic hilum. The tumor was sandwiched between the middle hepatic vein, right hepatic vein and inferior vena cava. It was a very difficult case. We decided to perform a right partial hepatectomy. The second hepatic hilum where the right hepatic vein, middle hepatic vein joined the inferior vena cava was carefully isolated and protected to control bleeding. The Pringle maneuver was applied intermittently 4 times (total occlusion time 31 minutes). The tumor was completely removed. Five ml anhydrous ethanol was injected into the cut surface of the liver. The whole operation was breathtaking, but convalescence basically uneventful. Follow-up by Sep 2015 at age 71, he was alive with ongoing survival of 22 years.

The above 2 cases are very typical examples that liver cancer can be transformed from a "ferocious tiger" to become a "tame cat". The key is "a hunter's courage and his martial arts." i.e. whether the guiding anti-cancer ideology is correct and measures applied appropriate. Simply speaking, we should strategically not be cowered by it and tactically take it seriously in the treatment of liver cancer. Neither "fearlessness" nor "seriousness" is dispensable, as they play important roles in the fight against liver cancer.

However, we should avoid the 2 extremes, one is excessive fear before treatment and the other blind optimism when planning treatment.

Especially in the latter, at times, the "real tiger" was wrongly thought to be a "paper tiger". This misunderstanding had led to many failures.

4.3 Lung Metastasis Means the Disease is in a Late Stage, is not Entirely True

A malignant tumor transferred from one location to another or from one organ to another, is called metastasis. Metastases are often thought to be rapid progression of the tumor and a late stage manifestation with a short lifespan, no long suitable for surgery. But our experience is different. We feel lung metastasis from liver cancer, especially a solitary lung metastasis is not so frightening. One should not be pessimistic.

Mr. Shen (case 12) is one of the most successful cases in our series. He received left hemihepatectomy for a huge tumor 12 cm in diameter in Sep 1975 at age 60. Four years later, a metastasis, 5cm in size, in the upper lobe of the left lung was found. A left upper lobectomy of the lung was performed in Oct 1979. Pathology of the lung specimen was hepatocellular carcinoma. Since then, no recurrence or metastasis was noted. Follow-up by Oct 2015 at age 99, he remained well with ongoing survival of 40 years.

In our present series, there were 4 cases of lung metastases from liver cancer (case 8, 12, 28 and 42). They survived for 32, 40, 20 and 28 years after liver resection and pulmonary resection. Aside from these examples, there are additional cases but not included here, because their survival has not yet reached the arbitrary requirement of 20 years. These results suggest that metastasis from liver cancer does not necessarily imply a late stage of the disease. Some are salvageable or even curable. Therefore, we should not give up surgical or local treatment easily in a patient with pulmonary metastasis after liver resection. Of course not all patients with metastasis from liver cancer are suitable for surgery.

4.4　Do not Ignore the Value of Hepatic Artery Surgery in the Treatment of Liver Cancer

In the human body, only liver has two sets of blood supply, hepatic artery and portal vein. Coincidentally, in liver cancer hepatic artery and portal vein seem to have a clear division of labor. Hepatic artery mainly supplies the cancer and portal vein the liver. Therefore, when the hepatic artery is blocked, growth of the cancer will be inhibited without affecting liver function and survival. The principle of hepatic artery surgery i.e. hepatic artery ligation and cannulation followed by intra-arterial infusion chemotherapy, in the treatment of liver cancer is the same as that of Transcatheter arterial chemoembolization (TACE). Hepatic artery surgery is more aggressive and results are better than TACE. In our 88 cases, 8 were treated by hepatic artery surgery and obtained long-term survival. They were case 22, 38, 42, 43, 51, 55, 57 and 88 and survived 35, 29, 28, 28, 27, 26, 24 and 20 years, respectively. They were all still well and alive. Prolongation of a patient's life is due to interruption of nutrition to the tumor, resulting in decreased tumor cell vigor, inhibition and cessation of tumor growth and even reduction of tumor volume. In some patients tumor volume was reduced to be suitable for hepatectomy. A part of patients with the 2-step resection could achieve long-term and high-quality survival. However, this procedure is not widely adopted. The reasons are that it is relatively complex, postoperative management relatively tedious and duration of intra-arterial chemotherapy relatively lengthy. Usually, the duration is several months or even over a year. We feel surgeons should not only grasp the key of this procedure but also postoperative management details. Both physician and patient need to have enough patience and perseverance.

Hepatic artery surgery and the 2-step resection should be carefully evaluated before being implemented. Generally, both early and very late liver cancer is not suitable. Hepatic artery surgery is powerless in patients with advanced hepatocellular carcinoma, because of the abundant blood supply and formation of collateral circulation.

Hepatic artery ligation and TACE can also be used to control bleeding from a ruptured liver cancer.

4.5 Multi-Modality Therapy is the Developing Trend, but Surgical Resection is Absolutely Irreplaceable in the Comprehensive Treatment

With progress in medicine, treatment of liver cancer has evolved from a single mode to a variety of treatment modalities.

In the 1960's liver resection was almost the only valuable therapeutic modality. In the late 70's and the early 80's, treatment gradually developed into multi-modalities In addition to hepatectomy, a succession of hepatic artery ligation with catheterization, hepatic arterial interventional therapy, cryosurgery, anhydrous alcohol injection, microwave, radiofrequency ablation, external irradiation, internal radiation, Gamma Knife, immunotherapy, Traditional Chinese Medicine, targeted therapy, etc came into vogue. Individual or combined application of these greatly improved outcome, especially when surgical resection was not suitable. Long-term survival of some patients in this series was due to comprehensive treatment. In general, the more treatment modalities for HCC, the greater range of options and the better the outcome.

Ms. Zheng (case 42) was one of the most complicated cases in our series. Two big tumors 9cm and 6cm were separately located in the right lobe and left medial lobe as well as close to the 1st hepatic hilum. Met with this situation, almost everyone felt totally at lost and helpless. Surprisingly, both tumors reduced in size and AFP dropped from 580μg/L to 40μg/L. after a hepatic artery procedure (ligation and cannulation of the hepatic artery). Subsequently, in Feb 1988, both tumors were completely resected and AFP dropped to normal.

Six years later, liver cancer metastasized to the lung and mediastinum with re-elevated AFP. In Oct 1994 the 3rd operation, right upper pulmonary lobectomy and mediastinal metastasis resection were carried out. In Mar 2014, B-ultrasound again found 2 recurrent lesions in the liver. Radiofrequency ablation was applied to the lesions in Jun 2014 with complete tumor necrosis and AFP returned to normal again. Follow-up by Sep 2015 at age 75, she remained well with ongoing survival of 28 years.

Although treatment of liver cancer can be varied, hepatectomy or liver transplantation is not completely replaceable. Transcatheter arterial chemoembolization (TACE) is popular and easily performed, but the degree of blood flow blockage and anti-cancer effect are not superior to that of hepatic artery ligation and cannulation. Furthermore, lethality to the cancer is far less than resection. Radiofrequency ablation and other local treatments are very lethal, but indication too limited to be widely used. The following: size, number, location, depth of tumor and distance from big blood vessels or bile duct need to be considered. Although both Chinese and Western anticancer medications are constantly being updated and administered, their effect is too weak to play a leading role. Liver resection is still the optimal option for large cancer with cancer thrombus or those located close to the hepatic hilum.

With progress in anesthesia, application of a variety of surgical instruments, including laparoscopy and introduction of the humanized service concept, intensity and injury of the operation have been reduced gradually and pain greatly relieved. Hepatectomy is no longer a great fear to patients. At present, it is not realistic or wise to use other therapies in place of hepatectomy.

References

Lin TY, Lee CS, Chen KM. 1987. Role of surgery in the treatment of primary carcinoma of the liver. A 31-year experience. Br J Surg, 74(9): 839-842.

Sitzmann JV, Order SE, Klein JL, et al. 1987. Conversion by new treatment modalities of nonresectable to resectable hepatocellular cancer. J Clin Oncol, 5(10): 1566-1573.

Tang ZY. 2012. Metastasis of hepatic cancer. In: Gu JR (ed), Primary liver cancer. Hangzhou: Zhejiang University Press, Heidelberg: Springer, 367-398.

Zhou XD, Tang ZY, Yu YQ, et al. 1989. Hepatocellular carcinoma: Some aspects to improve long-term survival. Journal of Surgical Oncology, 41: 256-262.

陆继珍, 刘康达, 余业勤, 等. 1986. 人体肝细胞性肝癌血供的研究. 肿瘤, 6: 183-184.

马曾辰, 汤钊猷, 余业勤, 等. 1995. 原发性肝癌外科手术概念的更新和术后长期生存. 普外基础与临床杂志, 2 (1): 42-44.

Part V

Irregular Hepatectomy—the Mainstay Procedure in Liver Cancer Resection

5.1 Regular Hepatectomy

Early surgeons advocated the classic resection, i.e. regular hepatectomy or anatomic hepatectomy. They are left lateral lobectomy, left hemi-hepatectomy, right hemi-hepatectomy and right trisectionectomy.

Left lateral lobectomy refers to a hepatectomy on the left of the sagittal sinus, including segments Ⅱ and Ⅲ. Large vessels and bile ducts can be treated intrahepatically. Left hemi-hepatectomy is a hepatectomy on the left of the middle hepatic vein, including segments Ⅱ - Ⅲ - Ⅳ. The left portal vein, left hepatic duct and left hepatic vein can be treated inside or outside the liver. Right hemi-hepatectomy is a hepatectomy on the right of the middle hepatic vein, including the right anterior and posterior lobes, i.e. segments Ⅴ - Ⅵ - Ⅶ - Ⅷ. The right portal vein, right hepatic duct, right and short hepatic veins need to be treated extrahepatically before resection. Right trisectionectomy refers to resection of the whole right liver and the left medial lobe, i.e. segments Ⅳ - Ⅴ - Ⅵ - Ⅶ - Ⅷ. In addition to the right sided vessels, the middle hepatic vein would need to be resected.

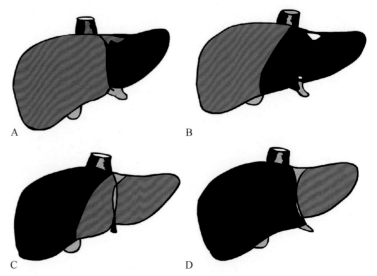

A   B

C   D

Fig. 5.1 The 4 classic regular or anatomic hepatectomies. (A) left lateral lobectomy, (B) left hemi-hepatectomy, (C) right hemi-hepatectomy and (D) right trisectionectomy

To avoid unnecessary sacrifice of normal liver tissue, hepatic segmentectomy is suggested to treat a small tumor, including single or multi-segmentectomies. These procedures also belong to the category of regular hepatectomy.

5.2   Irregular Hepatectomy

In general, the left liver accounted for one third of the total volume of the liver, the right liver two thirds. Similarly, about two-thirds of liver cancer is located in the right lobe. Irregular hepatectomy is a tumor-centered liver resection. In other words, it is performed neither according to the anatomic boundaries of the liver lobe or liver segment, nor vascular distribution in the liver. Irregular hepatectomies include subtotal resection of the right liver, partial resection of the left or right liver and wedge resection. It's advantages are: ① improved operative safety and avoided unnecessary sacrifice of normal liver parenchyma; ② no need to worry about blood supply disturbance and necrosis of the remaining liver; ③ short and long-term survival outcome not affected; ④ increase chance of resection in patients with cirrhosis who could not tolerate massive tissue loss in regular hepatectomy.

One of the recent advances in liver cancer surgery is irregular hepatectomy and it has become the mainstay procedure.

Of the 63 cases in our series, the tumor was solitary in 61 and underwent only a simple single resection. Among the 61 cases, 40 were in the right liver, 20 in the left liver and 1 in the middle lobe. Irregular hepatectomy accounted for 93% (37/40) of procedures performed for cancer in the right liver, 18% (4/20) in the left liver and 1 in the middle lobe. Totally, irregular hepatectomy in the left, right and middle lobes accounted for 69% (42/61) of resections. Two cases each had 2 tumors in the liver. One patient received a regular left lateral lobectomy and an irregular partial resection of the left medial lobe. The other patient underwent irregular partial resection of both right and left lobes.

5.3 Application of Lip-Shaped Hepatectomy in Irregular Hepatectomy

The lip-shaped incision in irregular hepatectomy is designed with the tumor at the center. The main points are: ① a lip-shaped incision with pointed ends at each end. It facilitates closure of the hepatic cut surface after removal of the tumor and reduces bleeding; ② traction on the preset sutures on both sides of the contemplated site facilitates making of the incision on normal liver tissue; ③ lifting the preset sutures will minimize contact with the tumor and squeezing it during the procedure; ④ it facilitates checking whether there is active bleeding and bile leak after removal of the tumor; ⑤ the pointed ends are most important in avoiding dead space formation when the hepatic cut surface is closely coapted and sutured.

Lip-shaped hepatectomy as an irregular hepatectomy has its unique features.

This procedure not only emphasizes the non-touch tumor technique to ensure a good outcome in patients with liver cancer. It also broadens indications and enhances safety of the resection.

How to deal with the hepatic cut surface directly affects safety of the operation. We prefer to close the cut surface rather than leaving it open. If the cut surface cannot be fully closed, we will partially close it but closely coapt and suture the deepest part as much as possible. The 2 sides of the cut surface are coapted with a large curved round needle using a thick silk suture or the special "liver suture".

Some surgeons worry closure of the hepatic cut surface could have adverse consequences. There is no need to worry about partial liver necrosis, because the liver is rich in blood supply. When suturing close to the first hepatic hilum, care should be taken to avoid iatrogenic biliary obstruction. When the stitch is tied with moderate strength, hepatic tearing could be avoided. In fact, a small hepatic tear is not serious.

Dealing with the hepatic cut surface varies from patient to patient. It should be coapted and sutured as much as possible to avoid complications due to inadequate or imperfect closure. There is no need to worry about bleeding from the cut surface and other complications when a lip-shaped hepatectomy is adopted.

Years ago, we encountered 2 patients who had massive bleeding from the hepatic cut surface. Closure of the hepatic cut surface is the best way to obviate this tragedy. Of course, how to deal with the cut surface varies with the surgeon's personal habit. If blood vessels and bile ducts on the cut surface were sutured and tied, bleeding and bile leak could be completely avoided. If the resection is not clear cut or clean and the cut surface treated only with hemostatic gauze or medical glue, complication is unavoidable.

Of the 63 cases in our series, 44 underwent 46 irregular hepatectomies, of which 2 cases each had 2 tumors. All of these irregular liver resections were performed with the so called lip-shaped hepatectomy.

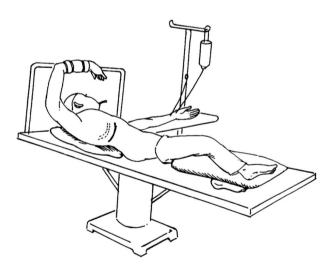

(A) Operative posture. The left arm extends horizontally, the right side is elevated (30°-45°) with cushion and right arm suspended

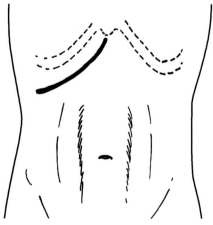

(B)The right subcostal incision

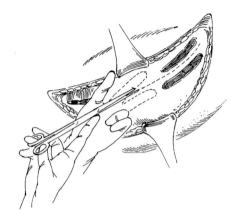

(C) the abdominal muscle and peritoneum being opened

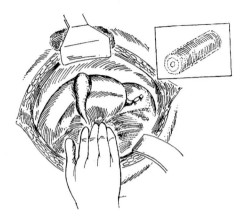

(D) Lift the rib cage up with the special "liver retractor". Pack the bowel away with rolled-up large pads to expose the liver and cancer

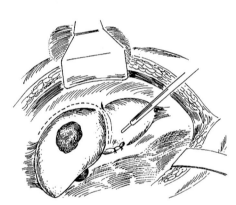

(E) The round, falciform and right coronal ligaments severed

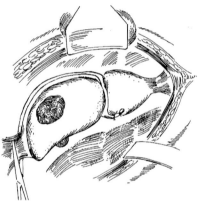

(F) Sever the right triangular ligament

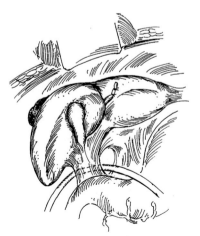

(G) Rubber tubing placed behind the hepatoduodenal ligament for first hepatic hilum occlusion

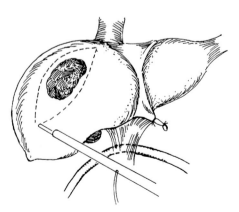

(H) Lip-shaped hepatic resection with tumor at the center and cautery marking the contemplated incision

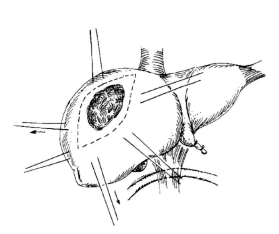

(I) Place sutures on both sides of the tumor for traction to avoid and minimize direct contact with the tumor

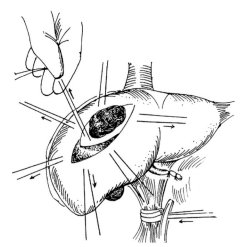

(J) Tumor removed with first hepatic hilum occluded. All vessels ligated or sutured individually

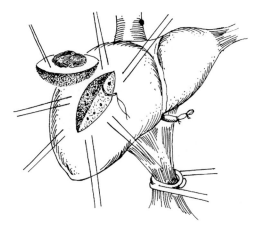

(K) Search for bleeding and bile leak on the cut surface after tumor removal

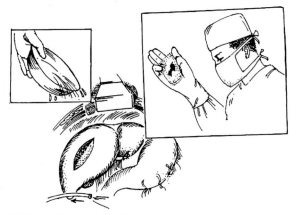

(L) Search for bile leak with dry gauze after flushing of the cut surface

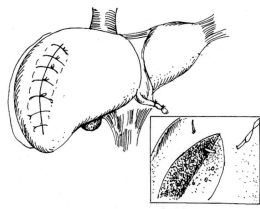

(M) Hepatic cut surface closely coapted and sutured to avoid formation of dead space. Avoid tearing of the liver when tying

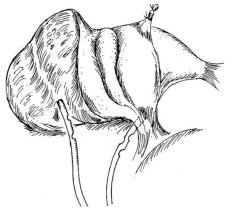

(N) Rubber tube drains placed under the right diaphragm and under the liver, or only under the right diaphragm

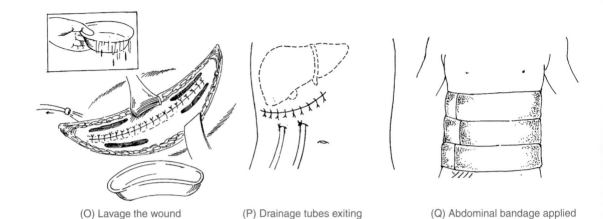

(O) Lavage the wound

(P) Drainage tubes exiting
separately

(Q) Abdominal bandage applied

Fig. 5.2　Lip-shaped hepatectomy

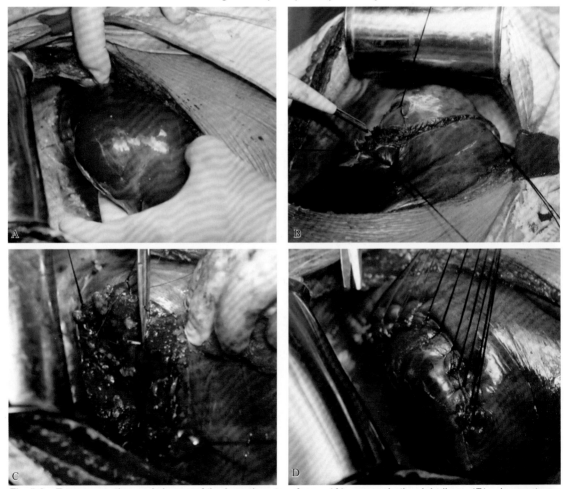

Fig. 5.3　Tumor resection and closure of the hepatic cut surface. （A）cancer in the right liver, （B）place sutures on both sides of the tumor, （C）suture bleeding points and bile leak on the cut surface and. （D）hepatic cut surface coapted and sutured

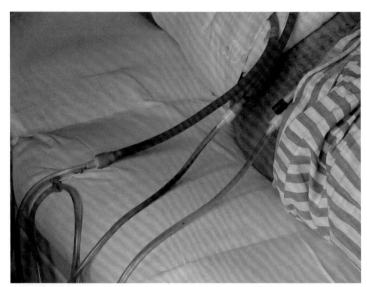

Fig. 5.4   Drainage tubes connected to collecting bags, negative pressure not required

5.4   Left Regular and Right Irregular Principle

Technically, left lateral lobectomy and left hemihepatectomy are not complex and sacrifice of normal liver tissue not great. Therefore, it is not necessary to use irregular hepatectomy for cancer in the left liver. We should tailor the procedure to suit the specific situation when performing either regular or irregular hepatectomy.

Our principle is "left regular and right irregular" in resection of liver cancer, i.e. regular resection preferred for cancer in the left liver and irregular resection in the right liver. However, the above principle should only serve as a reference guide.

5.5   Irregular Hepatectomy is Particularly Suitable for Liver Cancer at the Hepatic Hilum

Liver cancer at the hepatic hilum refers to those located less than 1 cm from the first, second or third hepatic hilum.

Liver cancer at the hepatic hilum is often located in segments Ⅳ, Ⅴ, Ⅶ or Ⅷ. Not all liver cancer located in segments Ⅳ, Ⅴ, Ⅶ or Ⅷ is called liver cancer at the hepatic hilum. Liver cancer in the above segments, but superficial or far from large vessels is not considered cancer at the hepatic hilum and resection is quite easy. Liver cancer in the caudate lobe i.e. segment Ⅰ is tightly wedged between the portal vein and inferior vena cava, absolutely belongs to a typical hepatic hilum liver cancer.

Most liver cancers with tumor thrombi in the main branches and trunk of the portal vein, main branch and trunk of the bile duct, trunk of the hepatic vein, or extending into the inferior vena cava also belong to the category of hepatic hilum liver cancer.

Liver cancer at the hepatic hilum is neither uncommon nor a contraindication to surgical resection.

Those in the right liver is often treated with irregular hepatectomy.

Of the 88 patients in our series, at least 8 were at the hepatic hilum. Four were located in the right liver and treated by irregular hepatectomy. The other 4 in the left liver received regular hepatectomy.

A good or even excellent outcome could be obtained in liver cancer at the hepatic hilum in the right liver if the surgeon performed a lip-shaped hepatectomy and paid special attention to the non-touch tumor technique with minimal direct contact or squeezing of the tumor.

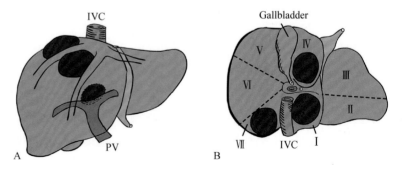

Fig. 5.5　Liver cancer at the hepatic hilum.（A）diaphragmatic view.（B）ventral view

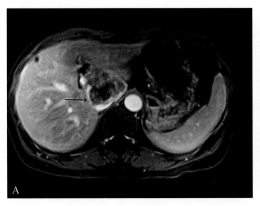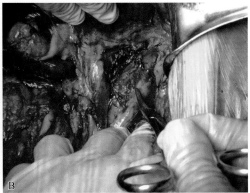

Fig. 5.6   Caudal lobe resection. （A）MRI Showing caudate lobe tumor wedged between the portal vein and inferior vena cave. （B）inferior vena cava at tip of the clamp after tumor removal

5.6   Positive Evaluation of the Hepatic Hilum Occlusion Technique in Hepatectomy

Hepatic hilum occlusion is one of the important technical links in liver resection. Hepatic hilum occlusion refers to occlusion of the first hepatic hilum i.e. the Pringle maneuver. Bleeding, especially massive breeding, in hepatectomy is at the root of all evils. Hepatic hilum occlusion can reduce bleeding during hepatectomy, especially in irregular hepatectomy. There are various ways to occlude the first hepatic hilum. We often use a rubber tube or catheter to loop around the hepatoduodenal ligament containing the portal triad. Once the loop is tightened, it can greatly reduce bleeding from the hepatic cut surface. Usually intermittent occlusion is applied. Each occlusion lasts 10-20 minutes with a 3-5 minutes free flow interval when multiple occlusions required. If the patient has no cirrhosis, occlusion time can be relatively longer. We have had experience of intermittent occlusion with a total occlusion time of 70-80 minutes.

With improved surgical technique, almost all liver resection could be performed by a right or bilateral subcostal incision and occlusion of the first hepatic hilum. A thoracoabdominal incision has now been abandoned.

The most serious consequence of bleeding is hemorrhagic shock and death. Even if it is not lethal, it impedes liver function recovery and convalescence.

The patient's life is safeguarded as long as bleeding is not excessive. Misconception in this area is "rather bleed and not be liver ischemic". The mistaken belief is that post-op liver failure is caused by hepatic hilum occlusion. We have used hepatic hilum occlusion for hundreds of times, and had not met with hepatic failure. Our principle is "occlusion for safety" and "occlusion for convalescence".

Hepatic hilum occlusion can be active or passive. In order to shorten operation time, an experienced surgeon can skillfully perform liver cancer resection without the occlusion. But for the majority of less experienced surgeons, if occlusion is not used a breathtaking scene of massive haemorrhage can usually be encountered. If that occurs it would be too late to use the occlusion and massive bleeding could cause adverse consequences. If the surgeon applied occlusion before hand, the above disastrous result could be avoided. Therefore, we advocate active hepatic hilum occlusion.

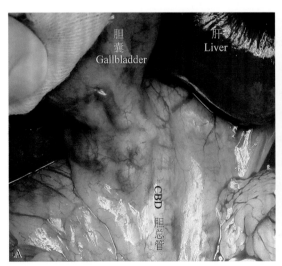 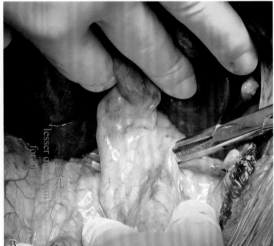

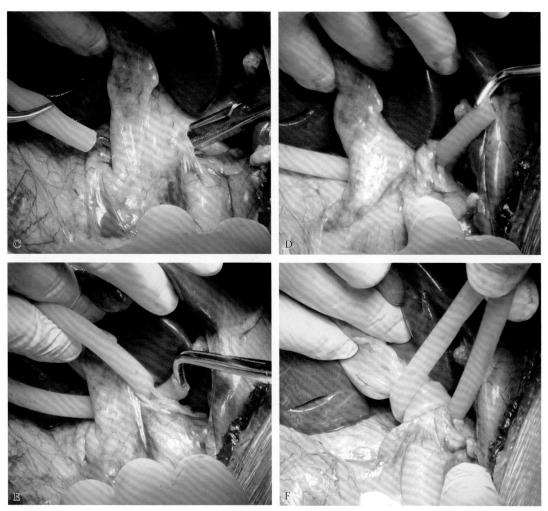

Fig. 5.7   Technique of hepatic hilum occlusion. (A) adequately expose the hepato-duodenum ligament by separating the lower edge of the liver and stomach. (B) partially sever the hepato-gastric ligament and place a Kelly clamp behind the hepato-duodenum ligament. (C)and (D)place a rubber tube behind the ligament.(E) and (F) Loop the rubber tube around the HD ligament and tighten it when needed

5.7   The Concept of Radical Resection in Liver Cancer is Different from Other Solid Tumors

In general, for a solid tumor, in addition to intact and complete resection, radical means a sufficient safety margin and total resection of the lymph nodes prone to be invaded.

However, in liver cancer only intact and complete tumor resection is adequate. A sufficient safety margin and removal of regional lymph nodes are not necessary.

Liver cancer in the caudate lobe, as the lobe clings to the inferior vena cava, is a typical liver cancer at the hepatic hilum. The inferior vena cava should be well protected. As the tumor is resected completely and intact outside the capsule, the procedure is still considered radical resection.

The above differences are mainly determined by the hepatic anatomy and biologic characteristics of liver cancer. Hepatic blood supply is very rich. In order to protect the blood vessels and bile ducts, especially the large vessels, radical resection need not and cannot require a sufficient safety margin.

In clinical practice, metastasis to the hepatic hilum lymph nodes is very rare in hepatocellular liver cancer. There is no need to resect the hepatic hilum lymph nodes.

In general, therapeutic outcome of a radical resection is better than that of palliative resection. But not all radical resections could obtain a curative effect. There is still the possibility of recurrence. However, occasionally, a palliative resection could surprisingly achieve a curative effect.

A genuine radical resection can only be validated on follow-up.

In fact, the curative effect of liver cancer surgery not only depends on the patient's condition, but also the surgeon's expertise of non-touch technique and avoiding queezing the tumor as well as close follow-up and additional treatment when needed.

5.8 One Must Balance Outcome and Operative Risks

We should always firmly put a patient's interests as our prime goal and not blindly pursue surgical outcomes without considering the risks of surgery.

In the early days of liver surgery, death due to hepatectomy was quite often, with a mortality of 20%−50%. The main causes of death were bleeding and liver failure. As experience accumulated and surgical skill improved, mortality greatly decreased. At present, in the hands of an experienced liver surgeon, mortality of hepatectomy is no higher than 1% and serious complications no higher than 10%. With this standard, the risks and costs of hepatic surgery is significantly decreased.

For every death due to hepatectomy for liver cancer, one must seek the cause and summarize the experience and lesson learned. If death is due to liver failure, one need to reflect whether the surgical indication has been carefully ascertained, especially the extent of cirrhosis in resection for a small liver cancer. If death is due to bleeding one need to reflect whether surgical skills in the management of large, deeply seated or hepatic hilum-located blood vessels as well as the cut surface need to be improved. If death is not due to bleeding or liver failure one need to reflect whether the patient's ability to respond to the stress of major surgical trauma and anesthesia had been overestimated. If surgical experience is insufficient, consultation with an experienced surgeon is needed. The experience of any single surgeon is limited. The patient will pay a heavy price if the surgeon is overconfident of his/her personal experience.

5.9   Suggestions to Reduce Mortality

5.9.1   Strict Control of Surgical Indications

The stress of undergoing hepatectomy is not only from trauma of the resection. General anesthesia and 2−3 days of early post-op fasting are also contributory. Function of the patient's heart, lungs, kidneys and digestive tract, etc. are also usually impaired in an aged and frail patient with comorbidities. Indications of liver resection should be even more tightly controlled.

Surgeons should never introduce only successful experiences of hepatectomy. The goal with the pros and cons of surgery, the risks and costs that could occur should also be made known to the patient. A comprehensive preoperative assessment is of utmost importance. A wrong decision due to inadequate assessment would lead to adverse consequences that could be very serious and difficult to rectify.

5.9.2 When Considering Surgery, do not Ignore the Impact of Age on Safety

In the past, people rarely lived to 70. Today, with improved living conditions, it is not surprising to live over 80. However, caution should be exercised in patients over 80. We should not only assess the patient's physical condition, but also consider the patient's ability to respond after a major stress.

At present, everyone wishes to prolong his/her life, live happily and enjoy old age in peace. If surgical outcome shortens life or impairs quality of life, and is expensive, we should not risk surgery.

In the past, patients with liver cancer did not live more than 3-6 months. It is because they were diagnosed late and already in an advanced stage. Today, with early diagnosis, their life has been extended to years. Moreover, there are more treatment options to choose from. Do not think surgery is the only treatment.

The risk of surgery in the aged is mainly due to their ability to respond to major stress is impaired. Even without surgery, the possibility of sudden death is increased, let alone the stress of trauma of liver surgery. The main causes of death in the aged are cardiopulmonary and/or systemic multiorgan failure.

The key to reduce mortality is to make a comprehensive pre-op assessment. When the assessment is neglected or inadequate, adverse consequences can be expected and no matter how successful or perfect the surgery is, a good outcome could hardly be achieved. In the aged, choosing a specialized or large hospital with experienced surgeons would be preferable, relatively safer and more effective. However, limited by a patient's difficulties, implementation of the above principle could be quite difficult.

5.9.3　Do not Think that Mortality of Small Liver Cancer is Very Low or Even 0

Since AFP was used in mass survey or screening of high-risk liver cancer subjects in China, many small and subclinical liver cancers were found and a very good outcome obtained. But it also made people blindly optimistic about its efficacy. In the past, we lacked understanding of the special feature of small liver cancer. The cancer is small because cirrhosis limited expansile growth of the tumor, but not its vitality. The proportion of small liver cancer with cirrhosis, especially severe cirrhosis, is higher than that of large liver cancer. Similarly, there is also a lack of understanding of the surgical risk of a small liver cancer in the presence of cirrhosis. One should not neglect consideration of the cirrhosis.

As experience accumulated, we have realized that we should not simply think that resection of a small liver cancer is only a minor procedure, operation easy, risk small and effect good. Never think that mortality of resection of a small liver cancer is zero. We recognized that the greatest risk of surgery is not necessarily those receiving the most difficult operation, but those undergoing the simplest liver resection with even minimal surgical bleeding. They do not die of bleeding but of postoperative liver failure.

When we decide on treatment of liver cancer, we are often asked by young doctors why we give up a minor resection of small liver cancer but proceed with a major resection for large or hilum-located liver cancer.

Our experience is that with a hilum-located liver cancer, although resection is of high risk, once a surgeon has mastered the precise skill to handle big blood vessels and avoided major bleeding, resection and convalescence could be more successful and satisfactory than expected. On the contrary, a small liver cancer resection can be dexterously and easily completed with minimal bleeding, unexpected trouble such as liver failure could ensue and even lead to death.

References

Bismuth H. 1982. Surgical anatomy and anatomical surgery of the liver. World J Surg, 6(1): 3-9.

Bismuth H, Houssin D, Castaing, et al. 1982. Major and minor segmentectomies "reglees" in liver surgery. World J Surg, 6(1): 10-24.

Fan J, Wu ZQ, Tang ZY, et al. 2001. Complete resection of the caudate lobe of the liver with tumor: Technique and experience. Hepato-Gastroenterol, 48: 808-811.

Iwatsuki S, Starzl TE. 1988. Personal experience with 411 hepatic resection. Ann. Surgery, 208(4): 421-434.

Lee NW, Wong J, Ong GB. 1982. The surgical management of primary carcinoma of the liver. World J Surg, 6(1): 66-75.

Okamoto E, et al. 1987. Current status of hepatic resection in the treatment of hepatocellular carcinoma. In: Okuda K, Ishak KG(eds), Neoplasm of the liver. Springer-verlag Tokyo, 353-365.

Starzl TE, Koep LJ, Weid R Ⅲ, et al. 1980. Right trisegmentectomy for hepatic neoplasms. Surg Gynecol Obstet, 150(2): 208-214.

Thompson HH, Tompkins RK, Longmire WP. 1983. Major hepatic resection: a 25-year experience. Ann Surg, 197(4): 375-388.

Wu MC. 1989. Experience in surgical resection of primary liver cancer. In: Tang ZY, Wu MC, Xia SS (eds), Primary liver cancer. Beijing: China Acad Publishers, Berlin: Springer-Verlag, 364-371.

Wu ZQ, Qiu SJ, Ma ZC, et al. 1999. An approach for difficult hepatectomy--retrograde hepatectomy in 29 patients with liver malignant tumor. Hepato-Gastroenterology, 46: 1140-1144.

Yu YQ, Tang ZY, Ma ZC, et al. 1991. Resection of the primary liver cancer of the hepatic hilus. Cancer, 67(5): 1322-1325.

Yu YQ, Tang ZY, Ma ZC, et al. 1993. Resection of segment Ⅷ of liver for treatment of primary liver cancer. Arch Surg, 128(2): 224-227.

陈孝平，吴在德，叶启发，等．1991．常温下阻断人肝血流行肝切除81例临床观察．中华外科杂志，29: 84.

第二军医大学第一附属医院肝外科．1977．特大肝脏海绵状血管瘤一例报告．中华外科杂志，15(1): 37-39.

马曾辰，汤钊猷，余业勤，等．2000．唇形切肝法用于原发性肝癌外科治疗．中国普外基础与临床杂志，7(1): 33-36.

马曾辰．2002．规则性与非规则性肝切除．见：严律南．肝脏外科．北京：人民卫生出版社，332-354.

马曾辰 . 2002. 提高肝癌手术安全性的若干问题 . 中国实用外科杂志 , 22(5):
  309-311.

彭淑牖 , 牟一平 , 彭承宏 , 等 . 1999. 肝尾叶切除术 26 例报告 . 中华外科杂志 ,
  37(1): 12.

孙惠川 , 钦伦秀 , 王鲁 , 等 . 2005. 术中美蓝试验可降低肝切除术后胆漏的发生
  率 . 中华外科杂志 , 43 (19) : 1291.

王成恩 . 1962. 有关肝切除问题的一些体会 . 中华外科杂志 , 10(10): 642-643.

王鲁 , 孙惠川 , 钦伦秀 , 等 . 2007. 肝癌解剖性肝切除的初步经验 . 中国普外基
  础与临床杂志 , 14(1)39-41.

吴志全 , 樊嘉 , 周俭 , 等 . 1998. 逆行肝脏部分切除术 . 中华外科杂志 , 36(9):
  533-535.

严律南 , 袁朝新 , 张肇达 , 等 . 1994. 应用半肝血流阻断行肝叶切除术 29 例报告 .
  中华外科杂志 , 32(1): 35-36.

杨甲梅 , 严以群 , 吴孟超 , 等 . 1997. 原发性肝癌行肝切除术后规则创面的处理 .
  中国实用外科杂志 , 17(4): 228-229.

余业勤 , 汤钊猷 , 周信达 , 等 . 1980. 低温无血切肝术一例报告 . 中华外科杂志 ,
  18(2): 146-147.

余业勤 , 汤钊猷 , 马曾辰 , 等 . 1989. 肝门区肝癌的手术切除 . 中华外科杂志 ,
  27(3): 157-159.

郑光琪 . 1998. 用肝门区域血管阻断法行肝段切除 202 例经验 . 中国实用外科杂
  志 , 18(3): 165-167.

周信达 , 程树群 . 1995. 肝切除术中肝血流阻断方法的评价 . 肝胆外科杂志 , 3: 8, 9.

Part VI

Hepatic Artery Procedure and the Two-Step Resection for Liver Cancer

With progress in science, technology and accumulation of clinical experience, treatment of liver cancer is becoming more and more diverse. It is generally accepted that surgical resection is the best treatment. However, there still are unsolved problems. They are: ① only a few liver cancer are suitable for surgical resection; ② the long-term result of surgical resection is not entirely satisfactory with a recurrence rate of greater than 50%; ③ some liver cancer resections are very traumatic with high risks. Thankfully, there are hepatic artery procedures in the treatment of liver cancer. Its advantages are: ① convert unsuitable for surgical resection patients to become suitable and extend survival; ② more excitingly, reduce volume of the cancer and make resection become with less risk; ③ decrease vitality and invasiveness of cancer cells with a relatively low recurrence rate. Hepatic artery therapy mainly refers to two kinds of methods, transcatheter arterial chemoembolization (TACE) and hepatic artery ligation with cannulation. Both treatments, especially the latter, compared with liver resection have the advantages of less bleeding and lower risk. Their therapeutic effects are obvious, sometimes even "miraculous", like the effect of "derive great power from a small generator".

The technique of hepatic artery procedures in detail and outcomes of the 20 patients subjected to this procedure will be discussed as follows.

6.1　Mechanism of Hepatic Artery Procedure in the Treatment of Primary Liver Cancer

Experimental and clinical practice have proved that nutrition of liver cancer, especially primary liver cancer, mainly comes from the hepatic artery. Interruption or decrease of blood supply from the hepatic artery will certainly affect survival of the cancer cells. Hepatic artery procedure is blocking blood flow in the hepatic artery by surgery and injecting chemical drugs via a catheter in the artery to kill the tumor as well as through starvation. Blood supply of the liver differs from other organs of the body. The liver is supplied by a dual blood supply, the hepatic artery and portal vein, while other organs have only the arterial route. Blood supply to the liver mainly comes from the portal vein, not the hepatic artery. However, blood supply to liver cancer is mainly from the hepatic artery, not portal vein. This means that hepatic artery occlusion does not or minimally affect viability of normal liver cells. Accordingly, hepatic artery ligation with cannulation or hepatic artery interventional therapy will obtain a good therapeutic effect on liver cancer with no deleterious effects on the normal liver.

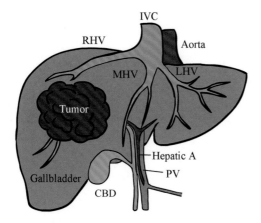

Fig. 6.1   Blood supply to the liver. Blood entering the liver: the portal vein (PV) and hepatic artery. Blood flowing out the liver: the right (RHV), middle (MHV) and left hepatic vein (LHV). Blood supply of primary liver cancer comes mainly from the hepatic artery and blood supply to the liver mainly comes through the portal vein

6.2   Hepatic Artery Ligation

Hepatic artery ligation is performed later than hepatic artery cannulation at our Hospital. The earliest hepatic artery ligation began in Feb 1968 at Zhongshan Hospital. In order to salvage a patient with massive hemorrhage from ruptured liver cancer, the surgeons were forced to stop the bleeding by ligation of the hepatic artery to tide over the difficulties. The successful treatment in this case suggested that in patients with liver cancer rupture, hepatic artery ligation can be performed if hepatectomy is beyond experience of the attending surgeon. Since 1974, we gradually carried out hepatic artery ligation for nonresectable liver cancer. At the beginning, only a branch of the hepatic artery was ligated, such as the right or left hepatic artery or their branch.

As experience accumulated, ligation of the main hepatic artery, such as the proper hepatic artery or common hepatic artery even both was carried out.

Ligation of the hepatic artery will reduce blood supply to the tumor and inhibit its growth. Generally, ligation of the hepatic artery can produce more direct effects on killing tumor cells than with drugs. At present, hepatic artery ligation is often combined with catheterization and subsequent intraarterial chemotherapy to achieve better results. Hepatic artery ligation can be performed when resection is difficult and/or with great risks and the desired outcome cannot be achieved.

One patient (case 55) received only right hepatic artery ligation. Amazingly, the tumor decreased from 10 cm to 2.6cm after 8 months. A hepatectomy was performed and he survived ongoing for 26 years.

6.2.1 Anatomy of the Hepatic Artery

For liver surgeons, hepatic artery ligation is not complicated. Hepatic artery is within the hepatoduodenal ligament on the left of the common bile duct and ventral to the portal vein. Hepatic artery consists mainly of 4 parts. They are the common hepatic artery, proper hepatic artery, right hepatic artery and left hepatic artery. The common hepatic artery originates from the celiac axis, courses along the superior border of the pancreas and bifurcates into the proper hepatic and gastroduodenal arteries near the pylorus. The proper hepatic artery ascends cephalad and branches into the right and left hepatic arteries near the hepatic hilum to supply the respective right and left liver. The right hepatic artery is generally 2–3cm in length longer, caliber larger than the left hepatic artery. Usually the proper hepatic artery is short, only about 1cm. There are many variations. Sometimes the proper hepatic artery is very short, or even "absent", with the common hepatic artery directly branching into the gastroduodenal, right hepatic and left hepatic arteries. Judgment of the hepatic artery and its branches is based on position, depth, caliber and course of the vessel. The gastroduodenal artery originates from the common hepatic artery, is slightly smaller than the hepatic artery and descends caudally dorsal to the duodenum. The right gastric artery usually comes from the common hepatic artery, sometimes from the proper hepatic artery. The right hepatic artery not infrequently arises from the superior mesentery artery and ascends cephalad dorsal to the common bile duct. On rare conditions, the left hepatic artery can arise from the left gastric artery and not the proper hepatic artery.

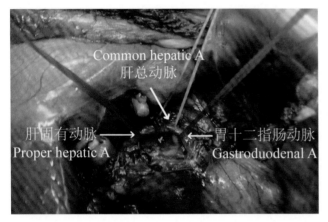

Fig. 6.2　Anatomy of the hepatic artery. The proper hepatic artery with a red, the common hepatic artery a yellow and the gastroduodenal artery a blue band

6.2.2　Ligation of the Hepatic Artery

If the surgeon placed the hepatoduodenal ligament between the left thumb and the other four fingers, pulsation of the hepatic artery could be felt and distinguish the common, proper, right or left hepatic artery. They can easily be dissected out. Ligation of the hepatic artery usually refers to simply ligation of the proper hepatic, common, right or left hepatic artery. The artery is usually ligated with a fine silk suture. In a right liver tumor, the advantage of ligation of the right hepatic artery is beneficial in reduction of the tumor mass. Its disadvantage is that collateral circulation to the tumor is easily established. In order to completely block blood flow, ligation of the right hepatic artery can be combined with ligation of the common and/or proper hepatic artery.

6.3　Hepatic Artery Cannulation

Hepatic artery cannulation was carried out in the treatment of liver cancer early in 1962 at Zhongshan Hospital. The cannulation procedure was very simple at that time. A fine plastic catheter was inserted through the right gastroepiploic artery and threaded into the proper hepatic artery. The catheter was fixed on the right gastroepiploic artery to prevent slipping out. The proximal end of the catheter was placed on the outside of the abdomen and clamped with a mosquito clamp. Standard intra-arterial chemotherapy was given. With the advent of hepatic artery ligation, simply hepatic artery cannulation has been abandoned. Details about hepatic artery cannulation will be described later.

Generally, simply hepatic artery cannulation and subsequent intra-arterial chemotherapy had certain beneficial effects on liver cancer. In the 1970s, due to lack of experience with hepatectomy, we performed simply hepatic artery cannulation with intra-arterial chemotherapy in a patient with liver cancer. After a few months, the tumor was controlled and resected. At that time, hepatic artery cannulation with intra-arterial chemotherapy won time for subsequent resection. As experience accumulated and technique improved, we no longer carry out simply hepatic artery ligation or simply hepatic artery cannulation but combined the two to maximize therapeutic results.

6.4   Hepatic Artery Ligation with Cannulation

Nowadays we rarely perform simply hepatic artery ligation or simply hepatic artery cannulation. These two procedures are often coupled together

At present, the operation is becoming more and more proficient. ① Dissect the hepatic hilum. The proper, common hepatic and gastroduodenal arteries are isolated. A catheter is inserted through the gastroduodenal artery into the proper hepatic artery under direct vision. In order to reduce bleeding, the catheter can also be inserted through the right gastroepiploic artery. But the disadvantage is the longer path increased difficulty of catheterization. ② Methylene blue is injected to confirm position of the catheter. ③ Tie the gastroduodenal and proper hepatic arteries around the catheter to prevent slippage. ④ Attach the end of the catheter into the port of a pump and place the pump subcutaneously in the abdomen to complete the procedure.

Variations of the right hepatic artery are not rare. The variant right hepatic artery originates from the superior mesenteric artery and is located on the right of the hepatoduodenal ligament dorsomedial to the common bile duct. When the right hepatic artery is not found in its normal position, existence of a variant right hepatic artery should be considered. The surgeon can feel pulsation of the variant right hepatic artery between the left index finger and thumb and a catheter inserted into the variant artery and tie around the catheter.

In order to prevent reflux of drugs into the right gastric artery and damage or even cause necrosis of the stomach, the right gastric artery must be ligated before initiation of intra-arterial chemotherapy.

6.5   Operation in Detail

Hepatic artery ligation with cannulation is a form of surgical treatment. The operation is performed in a surgical theater and under anesthesia. As the operation involves blood vessels, it has relative risks.

The procedure is as follows:

• A right subcostal incision, about 10cm in length is made.

• 2–3 pieces of large gauze pad are rolled up to pack away the intestines and greater omentum to fully expose the hepatoduodenal ligament.

• Dissect the cystohepatic triangle, disconnect the cystic duct, cystic artery and perform a cholecystectomy. The hepatic duct must be identified and protected before severing the cystic duct.

• The proper hepatic artery is isolated and follow the vine to get the melon. The common hepatic and gastroduodenal arteries are isolated. At times, the left and right hepatic arteries need to be dissected. Pay attention to protect the common bile duct, hepatic duct and portal vein.

• Fine silk sutures are looped around the gastroduodenal, common hepatic and proper hepatic arteries to control them in case of inadvertent bleeding.

• A fresh dilute heparin solution (1 ampoule 12,500 units heparin dissolved in 500ml of normal saline) is prepared.

• The dilute heparin solution is injected into the pump-catheter system to check for leakage.

• The catheter is soaked in liquid paraffin.

• A small segment of the gastroduodenal artery, about 1.5–2cm in length is isolated and ligated with fine silk suture.

• Make a small opening with a #11 scalpel in the gastroduodenal artery distal to the ligation and immediately insert the catheter to thread it to the proper hepatic artery and the relevant branch if needed. Then sever the artery and tie the ends. Be careful not to maneuver the catheter into the common hepatic artery.

Cannulation is the most important part of the procedure. It requires close cooperation between the surgeon and assistants.

• After insertion into the proper hepatic artery, the catheter should be fixed immediately with a fine silk suture to prevent slippage and bleeding.

• Diluted heparin is injected into the pump to check for obstruction.

• Methylene blue is injected to confirm precise location of the catheter. If the contemplated section of liver turns blue, confirms the catheter has reached the desired position.

• The proper hepatic and gastroduodenal arteries around the catheter are tied and blood flow blocked at the same time. Tying too tight will affect patency of the catheter, while too loose the catheter may slip out and cause bleeding.

• The pump is placed subcutaneously in the abdomen and fixed on the external oblique muscle aponeurosis with medium silk sutures.

• After closure of the abdominal incision, diluted heparin is again injected to reconfirm catheter patency.

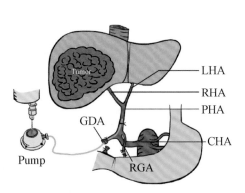

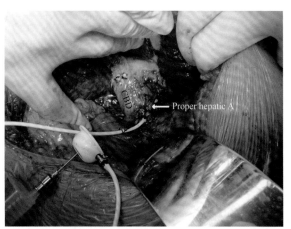

Fig. 6.3   Hepatic Artery Ligation with Cannulation. A catheter inserted through the gastroduodenal artery (GDA) to the proper hepatic artery (PHA). PHA tied around the catheter. Be careful not to maneuver the catheter into the common hepatic artery (CHA)

Fig. 6.4   Catheter inserted into the PHA through the GDA. PHA tied and catheter fixed

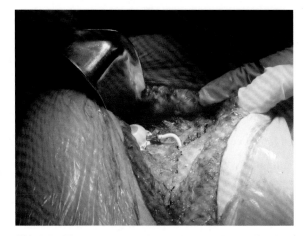

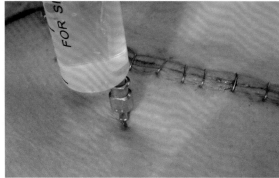

Fig. 6.5   The pump placed subcutaneously and fixed on the external oblique muscle aponeurosis with medium silk sutures

Fig. 6.6   Diluted heparin injected into the pump to reconfirm catheter patency after closure of the abdominal incision

6.6   The Embedded Pump-Catheter Infusion System

The embedded pump-catheter infusion system is also known as the

Implantable Access Port System.

Advantage of the pump-catheter system is that it maintains repeated intravascular therapy without affecting daily life of the patient.

The pump is buried in the abdomen subcutaneously. It can be repeatedly punctured to deliver drugs. There are two types of pump-infusion systems, one for intra-arterial and the other intravenous infusion. Difference between the two is mainly determined by pressure of the blood flow.

However, for hepatic intra-arterial therapy, either infusion systems can be used. At present, we use a German or US made intravenous infusion system.

The pump-catheter system mainly consists of two parts, the catheter and pump. A brief description of our commonly used products is as follows.

Catheter: 70cm in length, 1.6mm in outer diameter and 1.1mm inner diameter. It is made of polyurethane (PUR) and texture harder than silica gel. It is suitable for making wide lumen and thin walled catheters. The required length varies with the situation. The catheter and pump can be freely taken apart.

There are two types of catheter tip, slip-proof or simple. A slip-proof catheter prevents accidental removal, but relative resistance is slightly greater when inserting into the artery. A simple tip catheter is easier to insert. Once the ligature is tied, no need to worry about slippage.

The pump is composed of four parts: the body, diaphragm, base and the pump joint. The body is made of pure polysulfone, which is hard, non-allergenic and CT-compatible. The hard base can be pure polysulfone or titanium, 20–25mm in diameter. As long as the puncture position is accurate, no need to worry about the puncture needle penetrating the base. Capacity of the pump is about 0.33ml. With 1–2ml diluted heparin, the pump and catheter will be filled. The pump joint can be made of pure polysulfone or titanium. The membrane on the surface of the pump is made of high density silica gel. With a noninvasive needle, it can withstand 1,000–3,000 times of puncture. Diameter of the membrane is about 10mm. Technically, making a puncture within an area of 10mm is not very difficult. If met with difficulty, puncture under B-ultrasound guidance may be safer and more accurate.

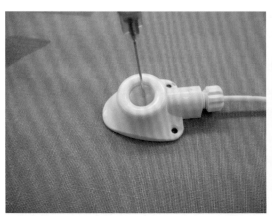
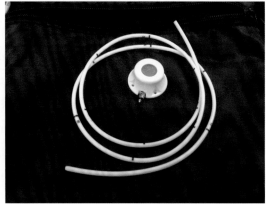

Fig. 6.7 The Embedded Pump-Catheter Infusion System. The pump is composed of four parts: the body, diaphragm, base and pump joint. The body is made of pure polysulfone. Capacity of the pump is about 0.33ml. The membrane on the surface of the pump is made of high density silica gel. With a noninvasive needle, it can withstand 1,000–3,000 times of puncture

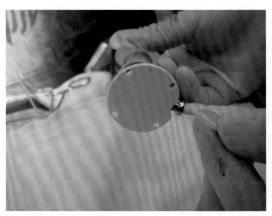
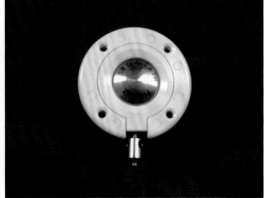

Fig. 6.8   The base can be pure polysulfone (left) or titanium(right). The texture is hard. As long as the puncture position is accurate, no need to worry about the puncture needle penetrating the base

6.7   Hepatic Intra-Arterial Chemotherapy via the Pump-Catheter System

The commonly used chemotherapeutic drugs are fluorouracil, cisplatin, and mitomycin. Fluorouracil is in solution. Cisplatin and mitomycin are powder and need to be dissolved in normal saline before use. The three drugs are 250mg, 20mg and 10mg per ampoule, respectively. The dosage of fluorouracil is 250mg or 500mg, cisplatin 20mg and mitomycin 10mg each time.

The treatment protocol is as follows: 1st day, fluorouracil 250mg, 2nd day, fluorouracil 250mg, 3rd day cisplatin 20mg and 4th day mitomycin C 10mg. The 4-day course of treatment is repeated every two weeks.

Usually, outcome would be best if treatment is continued for more than 3 months. If the patient is able to tolerate a larger double dose, the interval between courses can be extended to four weeks. The dosage of drugs as well as course of treatment can also be tailored to meet different situations.

The chemotherapeutic drugs are administered into the hepatic artery through the subcutaneous pump. The injection should be slow and each time should not be less than 3 minutes. Slow injection not only reduces pain, but also avoided the possibility of causing spread of the tumor. Slow injection can also reduce the risk of catheter slippage and bleeding.

Liver and kidney functions as well as blood count must be checked regularly, once a week, in the course of treatment.

Do not feel that puncture into the pump is a minor matter. It should be undertaken by an experienced physician to reduce complications, such as skin infection, necrosis, bleeding, catheter blockage and systemic infection.

The most important is to prevent trouble in the first place. It's better not to do anything than doing it wrongly.

An experienced physician can accurately and directly puncture through the abdominal skin into the pump with the special fine needle. Then diluted heparin and medications are injected indirectly into the hepatic artery. If the physician lacks the necessary expertise or the abdominal skin is too thick, it is better to puncture under type-B ultrasound guidance. After administration of the drugs, the catheter should be flushed with heparin.

It is best to puncture with the special fine needle or a #7 needle. Checking quality of the needle in advance is important. When a poor quality needle is used, it can cause membrane damage and bleeding.

Preparation of the heparin solution: 12,500U heparin is diluted in

100 ml of normal saline. The amount used to flush and seal the catheter is about 3–5ml each time.

At times, cisplatin can cause vomiting, but usually not serious. If vomiting is severe, antivoming drugs can be used in advance, for example, 0.3mg of Ramosetron Hydrochloride intravenously. Mitomycin must not be injected outside the pump, as it can cause skin necrosis and severe pain. Therefore, the needle must be punctured into the pump. When outside the pump, there is increased resistance, swelling of the skin and solution seeping through the needle puncture.

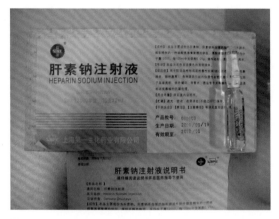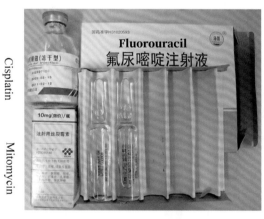

Fig. 6.9   Heparin sodium (left)and anticancer drugs (right). Preparation of the heparin solution: 12,500U heparin diluted in 100ml of normal saline. Anticancer drugs including Fluorouracil, Cisplatin, Mitomycin, etc.

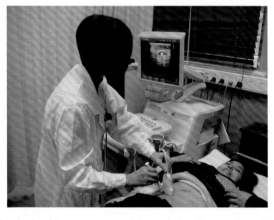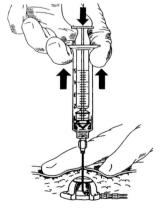

Fig. 6.10   A physician can accurately and directly puncture through the abdominal skin into the pump with the special fine needle. If the abdominal skin is too thick, the puncture may be performed under B-ultrasound guidance

6.8 Transcatheter Arterial Chemoembolization(TACE)

Transcatheter arterial chemoembolization (TACE) usually refers to transcatheter hepatic arterial chemoembolization. TACE is also commonly called hepatic artery interventional therapy.

The principle of TACE in the treatment of liver cancer is the same as that of hepatic artery ligation and cannulation with intra-arterial chemotherapy. Both are implemented via the hepatic artery. However, there is a great difference between TACE and hepatic artery surgery. ① Usually, TACE does not fall into the category of surgical treatment, but is performed by a radiologist, oncologist or digestive physician. ② TACE is performed in the interventional room with X-ray monitoring. A special sterile catheter is inserted selectively or superselective into the femoral artery at the groin, then through the iliac, abdominal aorta and celiac axis as conduit finally into the hepatic artery. ③ TACE is performed under local anesthesia and convalescence speedy. ④ Position of the catheter is displayed on the monitor and removed after treatment. ⑤ Hepatic artery occlusion by TACE is through embolization of a mixture of lipiodol and gelatin sponge rather than ligation of the artery. Degree and duration of the blockage are not as good as hepatic artery ligation. The chemotherapeutic drugs used are basically the same as in chemotherapy via the pump-catheter system. ⑥ Generally, only a single hospital stay is required in hepatic artery surgery. Repeated chemotherapy with the pump can be administered in the outpatient clinic. However, each TACE requires hospitalization. ⑦ Patients with arteriovenous fistulae are not suitable for TACE, but these fistulae do not affect hepatic artery surgery. ⑧ TACE can inhibit tumor growth, and a huge liver tumor might be reduced to meet the requirement for a 2-step resection (Case 20). TACE can prolong survival, but it is rare to have survival for more than 20 years.

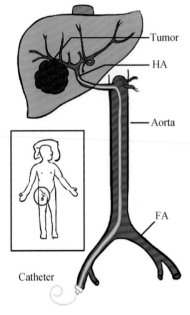

Fig. 6.11 Transcatheter arterial chemoembolization (TACE). A special sterile catheter inserted selectively or superselective into the femoral artery (FA) at the groin, then through the iliac, abdominal aorta and celiac axis as conduit finally into the hepatic artery (HA). Thereafter, chemotherapeutic drugs and embolic agents are injected

6.9   Two-Step Resection of Liver Cancer

Although both hepatic artery ligation with hepatic intra-arterial chemotherapy via the pump–catheter system and TACE can inhibit tumor growth, lead to necrosis and even tumor mass reduction, outcome is not necessarily fully satisfactory. There could be a missed fish out of the net. If this happened a subsequent surgical resection could probably greatly improve outcome. This is often referred to as a 2-step or 2-stage resection. We feel the 2-step resection is a good option when the outcome of hepatic artery surgery or TACE meets the expected requirement. At times, certain resectable tumors might also consider the 2-step resection to improve outcome and reduce risks.

The 2-step resection is equivalent to the strategy and tactic of "first encircle, then annihilate" the enemy to win a big victory.

In fact, for some patients, a reasonable and appropriate 2-step resection is better than blind resection. Technically, at present, there is almost no liver cancer that cannot be resected. However, outcome could be quite different. The long-term survival of large and extra large liver cancer receiving palliative resection is very low. If the surgeon augments pre-op evaluation awareness, forgoes blind palliative resection, institutes rigid comprehensive treatment, and appropriately employs a 2-step resection, the curative outcome of liver cancer and long-term survival would be greatly increased. Recommendation of an appropriate increase in the proportion of 2-step resection does not mean rejection of primary resection of liver cancer. This is simply a difference in opinion on the issue of extent of surgery. We strongly admonish against irrational high-risk excessive resection.

However, merits of the 2-step resection should not be overestimated. Liver cancer is a stubborn and prone to recur disease. Patients undergoing the 2-step resection should still be followed closely to detect and treat recurrence and metastasis.

With regard to selection of TACE and hepatic artery surgery, we tend to choose TACE first. The reasons are: A) Technically, TACE is easy and carried out nation wide. B) There is no major surgical trauma. However, hepatic artery surgery has unique advantages: ① hepatic artery ligation induced vascular occlusion is far more complete than TACE; ② the hepatic, right gastric and gastroduodenal arteries are ligated, greatly reduced side effects due to reflux of drugs; ③ inject drugs through the pump is convenient. With care, repeated treatment via the pump-catheter system can last 6 months to a year; ④ only drugs are injected without iodized oil and there is no need to worry about adverse effects from the arteriovenous fistulae. However, unfortunately hepatic artery surgery is not widely accepted. The reasons are: many doctors do not understand the value of hepatic artery surgery, the procedure of injecting drugs into the buried pump is tedious and relatively complex. Therefore, treatment choice should be tailored to suit specific circumstances and vary with the patient.

However, we should also remember that hepatic artery therapy is not a panacea. It is not effective for advanced liver cancer, and also not always ideal for treatable liver cancer. Effect of its treatment is determined by sensitivity and tolerance of tumor cells to "ischemia" and the drugs used. Experience and expertise of the clinician also are contributory. Hepatic artery surgery and TACE are not without complications and sometimes they cannot be completely avoided. In order to achieve the best outcome, physicians need to constantly sum up experience and improve expertise.

6.10 Typical Cases in Hepatic Artery Therapy

In this set of 20 patients, 9 patient (Patient 1-9) have been described in detail as they belong to the 88 case series. They have survived 20 or more years after hepatic artery surgery, either alone or supplemented with two-stage resection. Outcomes have been amazingly satisfactory.

Ten patients (Patients 10-19) in this set but not in the 88 cases series also had hepatic artery surgery. Outcomes were equally satisfactory. They were not included because their ongoing survival has not yet reached the arbitrary requirement of 20 years. However, these are later cases and their data, especially imaging findings are more complete. A trivial maneuver elicited manifold great effects. We strongly feel hepatic artery surgery should not be neglected as a low-risk minimal trauma treatment option when suitable conditions exist.

Transcatheter arterial chemoembolization (TACE) usually refers to transcatheter hepatic arterial chemoembolization. The principle of TACE is the same as that of hepatic artery ligation and cannulation with intra-arterial chemotherapy. Both are implemented via the hepatic artery. However, TACE dose not belong to the scope of surgical treatment. As for efficacy, TACE is not as good as hepatic artery surgery. But at times TACE can be quite effective and Patient 20 is a good example.

Illustrative cases as follows.

Patients 1-9 see cases 22, 24, 35, 38, 42, 43, 51, 55 and 57, in part Ⅰ.

Patient 10 (No. 320532)

Mr. Qiu, liver cancer ongoing 17 years survival after hepatic artery surgery and 2-step resection.

He was explored in Apr 1998 at age 42. A huge tumor 12cm was located in segments Ⅵ - Ⅶ of the liver, close to the IVC. Diagnosis by needle biopsy was HCC. Hepatic artery surgery, ligation and cannulation of the proper hepatic artery with ligation of the common hepatic artery was carried out. Post-op intra-arterial chemotherapy was given. Four months later, the tumor reduced to 6.5cm, AFP dropped from 553μg/L to 181μg/L. In Aug 1998, a 2-step resection right partial hepatectomy was performed and the subcutaneous pump-catheter system was also removed. Texture of the tumor specimen was hard with massive necrosis. After resection, AFP dropped to normal. Follow-up by May 2015 at age 58, he was alive and well.

Patient 11 (No. 341921)

Mr. Xiao, liver cancer ongoing 15 years survival after hepatic artery ligation and cannulation with 2-step resection.

He was explored in Sep 1999 at age 44. A tumor 8 cm with unclear boundary was located in segments Ⅵ – Ⅶ of the liver close to the major vessels. His liver was moderately cirrhotic. Diagnosis by needle biopsy was HCC. Hepatic artery surgery, ligation of the common and proper hepatic arteries and cannulation of the proper hepatic artery with intra-tumor anhydrous ethanol injection were carried out. Six months later, the tumor reduced to 2/3 of its original size with clear boundary. In Mar 2000, a 2-step resection right partial hepatectomy was performed. The tumor specimen was hard, 6cm in size with extensive necrosis. Pathology was grade Ⅱ-Ⅲ differentiated HCC. AFP dropped from 553μg/L to normal. Follow-up by May 2015 at age 58, he was alive and well with ongoing tumor-free survival of 15 years.

Patient 12 (No. 354970)

Mr. Zheng, liver cancer 10 years survival after hepatic artery surgery and 2-step resection.

He had 2 surgeries for liver cancer. The first was in Jul 2000 at age 48. A 16cm huge tumor was located in the middle and upper part of the right lobe with no liver cirrhosis. Diagnosis by needle biopsy was HCC. Ligation with cannulation of the proper hepatic artery and ligation of the common hepatic artery as well as intra-tumor anhydrous ethanol injection were carried out. Fluorouracil, cisplatin and mitomycin intra-arterial chemotherapy was given. After 4 months imaging found the tumor reduced significantly in size and AFP dropped from 3,409μg/L to 162μg/L. In Nov 2000, the 2nd operation was performed. The huge tumor had reduced in size and appeared as 2 separate lesions 10 and 2.5cm tumors close to each other. A 2-step resection right subtotal hepatectomy was performed. Post-op convalescence was smooth and AFP dropped to normal. Pathology showed necrosis accounted for 90%

of the tumor specimen with no viable tumor cells. The patient soon went back to work.

As the operation was successful and convalescence smooth, he was busy with his work, became over optimistic about his outcome and neglected regular follow-up. Regretfully, he died of recurrence at age 58 in Oct 2010, the 10th post-op year.

Patient 13 (No. 138489)

Mr. Liu, liver cancer ongoing 12 years survival after hepatic artery surgery and 2-step resection.

He had 2 surgeries for liver cancer. The first was in Feb 2003 at age 46. A 15cm huge tumor occupied almost the entire right lobe of the liver. Diagnosis by needle biopsy was HCC. Ligation with cannulation of the right hepatic artery and ligation of the common hepatic artery as well as cholecystectomy were carried out. Fluorouracil, cisplatin and mitomycin intra-arterial chemotherapy was administered. After 6 months, AFP dropped from 46.6μg/L to 3.2μg/L and tumor size decreased significantly. In Aug 2003, at the 2nd operation the tumor had reduced to 9cm with a clear boundary. A right partial hepatectomy was performed. Gross and microscopic examination showed 90% of the tumor was necrotic. Convalescence was smooth and he soon returned to work. Follow-up by May 2015 at age 57, he was alive and well with ongoing survival of 12 years.

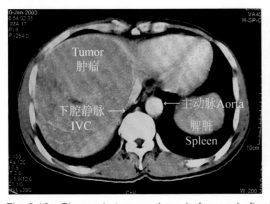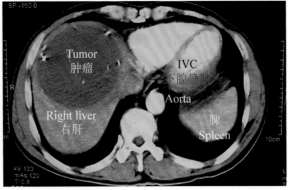

Fig. 6.12   Change in tumor volume before and after hepatic artery surgery. Left: a 15cm tumor in the right lobe close to the IVC (pre-op CT, Jan 30 2003). Right: tumor significantly smaller and further away from the IVC with extensive tumor necrosis. (After hepatic artery surgery, CT Mar 2003)

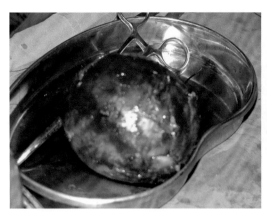 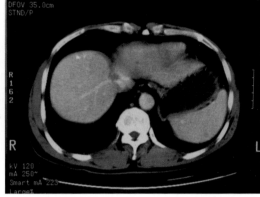

Fig. 6.13   Liver cancer specimen and post-op CT. Left: a 6 cm tumor specimen with hard texture and massive necrosis. Right: CT (Mar 2006) showing liver regeneration at operated site with no new lesion

Patient 14 (No. 142282)

Mr. Zheng, liver cancer ongoing 11 years survival after hepatic artery surgery and 2-step resection.

He had 2 surgeries for liver cancer. The first was in Dec 2003 at age 53. An 11cm huge tumor was located in the right postero-superior part of the liver close to the IVC. Diagnosis by needle biopsy was HCC. Ligation with cannulation of the proper hepatic artery and cholecystectomy were carried out. Intra-arterial infusion chemotherapy was given. After 8 months, AFP dropped from 146.8μg/L to 68.8μg/ L with reduction in tumor size. In Aug 2004 at operation, the tumor had reduced to 8cm with a clear boundary. A right hepatectomy was performed and he recovered uneventfully. AFP returned to normal.

Follow-up by May 2015 at age 64, he was alive and well with ongoing survival of 11 years.

Patient 15 (No. 539768)

Mr. Zhang, liver cancer ongoing 8 years survival after hepatic artery surgery and comprehensive treatment.

He had hepatic artery surgery with post-op comprehensive treatments for primary liver cancer and achieved a good outcome.

The first operation was in Oct 2007 at age 67. A 6cm tumor

was located in the right lobe, but associated with severe cirrhosis. Diagnosis by needle biopsy was HCC. After full onsite assessment, ligation with cannulation of the proper hepatic artery was carried out. Intra-arterial fluorouracil chemotherapy was given. After 2 months, B ultrasound showed the tumor had reduced in size with no arterial blood flow. Follow-up on Dec 2009, the patient was in good condition. B-ultrasound and CT showed the tumor had reduced to 3 cm with no visible blood flow, denoted tumor necrosis. Unfortunately, in Oct 2010, MRI found 2 new lesions, one in the left lobe and the other in the right lobe. In Nov 2010, radiofrequency ablations were administered to the recurrent lesions. In Dec 2011, a 2nd radiofrequency ablation was applied to the lesion in the right lobe. His condition remained stable for more than 3 years. In Mar 2015, CT detected a 2 cm new lesion in the left lobe. Because he was in good physical condition, location and size of the tumor suitable for surgical resection, a left lateral lobectomy was performed in May 2015. The former right lobe tumor that underwent hepatic artery surgery had become a scar and the 2 lesions subjected to radiofrequency ablation were completely necrotic. The operation was basically smooth and convalescence uneventful. Pathology was HCC with nodular cirrhosis. Follow-up in Oct 2015, the patient was alive with ongoing survival of 8 years.

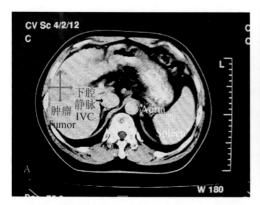 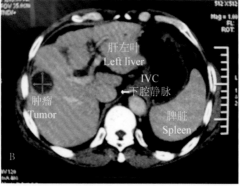

Fig. 6.14　Tumor size before and after hepatic artery surgery. A: Pre-op CT, a 6 cm tumor in the right lobe with severe cirrhosis (Sep 2007). B: Post-op CT, tumor reduced in size with necrosis and a clear boundary (Apr 2008)

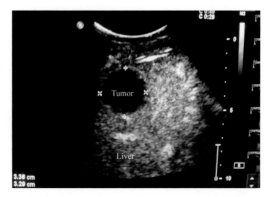

Fig. 6.15   Post-op contrast-enhanced B-ultrasound imaging. Three months after hepatic artery surgery, contrast-enhanced B-ultrasound imaging showed a hypoechoic mass with no contrast enhancement denoting tumor necrosis (Jan 2008)

Patient 16 (No. 605413)

Ms. Xia, liver cancer ongoing 6 years survival after hepatic artery surgery and 2-step resection as well as comprehensive treatments.

She had an AFP-negative liver tumor and was explored in May 2009 at age 59. A 13cm huge tumor was located in the right superior part of the liver. Diagnosis by needle biopsy was HCC. Hepatic artery surgery, ligation with cannulation of the proper hepatic artery and cholecystectomy were carried out. One year after intra-arterial chemotherapy, the tumor was significantly reduced in size. A 2-step resection right partial hepatectomy was performed in May 2010. The tumor was 8cm and necrosis exceeded 50%. Pathology was HCC with necrosis. Unfortunately, in Nov 2012, her condition suddenly deteriorated. B-ultrasound, chest X-ray and CT revealed recurrence in the right lobe, metastasis to the right lung and cancer thrombi in the IVC. Gamma Knife treatment and cinobufagin systemic chemotherapy via the right subclavian vein as well as orally were given. The above treatments yielded magical effects. In Mar 2014, chest and abdominal CT showed that almost all the above recurrences had disappeared. Follow-up by Jul 2015, the 6th post-op year, she had the same mental state, appearance and physical strength of a normal person. She could take care of herself, and do house work. The mechanism of action of cinobufagin on liver cancer deserves further in-depth study.

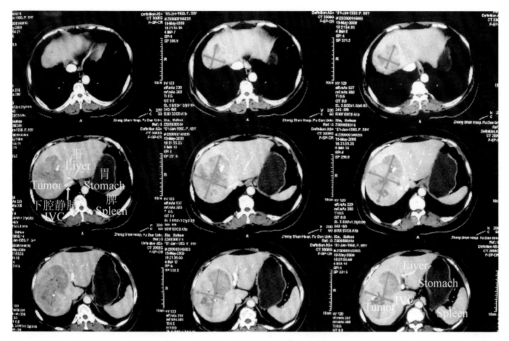

Fig. 6.16   A 13cm huge tumor close to the 1st and 2nd hepatic hilum. CT (May 19 2009) before hepatic artery surgery

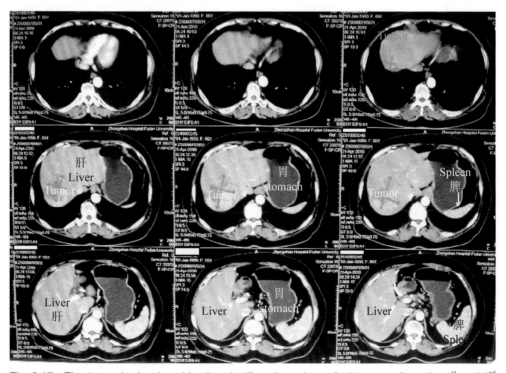

Fig. 6.17   The tumor had reduced in size significantly and was further away from the 1st and 2nd hepatic hilum. CT after hepatic artery surgery (Apr 21 2010)

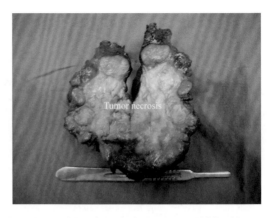

Fig. 6.18   Pathology of the resected specimen: HCC with exceeding 50% necrosis of the tumor. (May 2010)

Patient 17 (No. 647752)

Mr. Pan, liver cancer ongoing 5 years survival after hepatic artery surgery and comprehensive treatment.

He had a solid space-occupying lesion in the liver and AFP-negative. He was explored In May 2010 at age 41. A 3.5 cm tumor was located in the right lobe of the liver. Diagnosis by needle biopsy was HCC. Because of severe cirrhosis and mild coagulopathy, hepatic artery surgery, ligation and cannulation of the proper hepatic artery with intratumor ethanol injection as well as cholecystectomy were performed. The tumor gradually reduced in size. In Apr 2013, B ultrasound showed the tumor had decreased to 1.4cm without obvious blood flow.

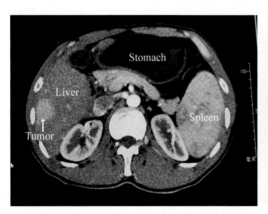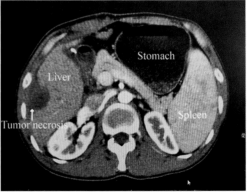

Fig. 6.19   Left: CT before hepatic artery surgery, a 3.5cm liver cancer with rich blood supply in the right lobe as well as severe cirrhosis and splenomegaly (May 13 2010). Right: CT after hepatic artery surgery, the tumor had a clear boundary without obvious blood flow denoting tumor necrosis. (Jun 30 2010)

However, in Oct 2014, enhanced CT showed a 1.8cm new recurrence in the left lobe with AFP elevated to 56.8μg/L. Radiofrequency ablation and subsequent TACE were administered. Follow-up by Jul 2015, he was stable with ongoing 5 years survival. He could take care of himself and do housework. Imaging examination revealed both lesions were necrotic and AFP normal.

Patient 18 (No. 744833)

Mr.Duan, liver cancer ongoing 3 years survival after hepatic artery surgery and 2-step resection

He was explored for a space-occupying lesion in the liver on B-ultrasound and CT with positive AFP in May 2012 at age 49. A 15cm huge tumor was located in segments Ⅴ-Ⅵ-Ⅶ-Ⅷ, close to the 1st hepatic hilum. Diagnosis by needle biopsy was HCC. Ligation and cannulation of the right hepatic artery and cholecystectomy were carried out. Post-op intra-arterial chemotherapy and oral Chinese Herbal Medicine were administered. Five months later, the tumor significantly decreased in size and was further away from the 1st hepatic hilum. AFP dropped from 1,390μg/L to normal. In Oct 2012, a 2-step resection right hemihepatectomy was carried out. The tumor had shrank to 8 cm with a hard texture and massive necrosis exceeded 80% of the tumor specimen.

Post-op convalescence was basically uneventful and his condition stable. Follow-up by May 2015, he was alive and well.

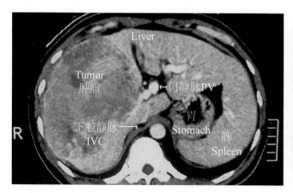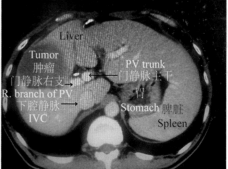

Fig. 6.20   CT before and after hepatic artery surgery. Left: pre-op CT: showing a huge tumor, 147mm x 95mm in the right lobe, close to the right portal vein (Apr 20, 2012). Right. post-op CT showing the significantly shrunken tumor with necrosis and further away from the 1st hepatic hilum (Aug 21, 2012)

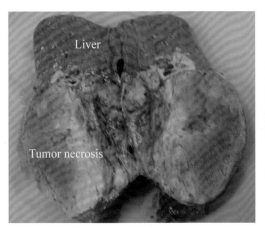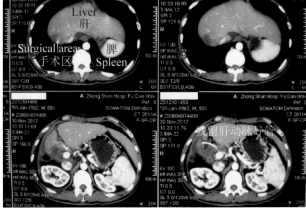

Fig. 6.21 Tumor specimen and post-op CT finding.Left: Tumor specimen with exceeding 80% necrosis of the tumor (2-step resection in Oct 2012). Right: CT one month after hepatic resection showing no residual tumor or new lesion at the operated site (Nov 30, 2012)

Patient 19 (No. 771663)

Mr. Zhou, liver cancer ongoing 3 years survival after hepatic artery surgery.

He had hepatitis history and a 26mm×22mm space-occupying lesion in the liver on B-ultrasound during physical check-up in Apr 2012, because the mass was small with negative AFP, he was closely followed. In Oct 2012, the tumor had increased to 35mm×31mm with characteristics of cancer on B-ultrasound, CT and MRI and AFP elevated to 112.9μg/L. Liver cancer was highly suspected. Due to poor cardiopulmonary function, hypertension and old age, hepatectomy would be of very high risk. The three treatment options were TACE, radiofrequency ablation and hepatic artery surgery. Exploration was performed in Nov 2012 at age 82 because the patient incessantly wished to have a definitive diagnosis. Liver cancer was confirmed. The tumor was 3.5cm located in the right posterior lobe with moderate cirrhosis. Cannulation of the proper hepatic artery and ligation of the common, proper and left hepatic arteries as well as cholecystectomy were performed. The procedure was smooth and convalescence uneventful. Post–op intra-arterial chemotherapy and oral compounded cantharidis capsules were administered. Intra-tumor blood flow was not visible on B-ultrasound 2 weeks after surgery. AFP decreased to normal at 1 month. Follow-up by Nov 2015 at age 85, the tumor had disappeared on B-ultrasound. He was alive and enjoying a happy old age life.

Patient 20 (No. 281548)

Ms. Zhou, liver cancer 17 years survival (Dec 1994–Jun 2011) after TACE and 2-step resection.

She had 4 TACEs for a 13cm huge liver cancer at the Shanghai Huadong Hospital from May 1994 to Oct 1994 and achieved a good result. Her tumor reduced to 6cm and AFP dropped from 790μg/L to 130μg/L. In Dec 1994 at age 63, a 2-step resection right partial

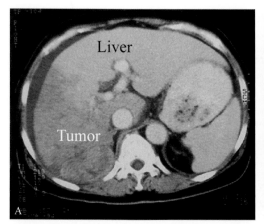
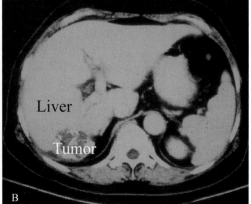

Fig. 6.22   CT before and after TACE. (A) pre-TACE CT: showing a 13cm huge tumor in the right lobe (May 7 1994); (B) post-TACE CT showing a 6cm significantly shrunken tumor (Oct 20, 1994)

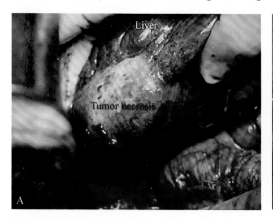
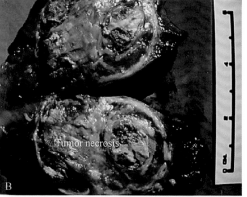

Fig. 6.23   Tumor at operation and resected specimen. (A) at operation the tumor had shrunken, texture hard and boundary clear. (B) tumor specimen: necrosis accounted for 90% of the tumor with thick and tough capsule

hepatectomy was performed at our hospital. The procedure was basically smooth and recovery uneventful. After resection, AFP dropped to normal. Pathology: necrosis accounted for 90% of the tumor with no viable tumor cells. No recurrence was found at 17 years on regular follow-up. Regretfully, in Jun 2011 at age 80, she died of cerebral infarction.

References

Friesen SR, Hardin CA, Kittle CF. 1967. Prolonged survivals of ten partial hepatectomies and second look procedures for primary and secondary carcinoma of the liver. Surgery, 61(2): 203-209.

Lin G. 1989. Selective angiography of primary liver cancer. In: Tang ZY, Wu MC, Xia SS (eds), Primary liver cancer. Beijing: China Acad Publishers, Berlin: Springer-Verlag, 297-304.

Sitzmann JV, Order SE, Klein JL, et al. 1987. Conversion by new treatment modalities of nonresectable to resectable hepatocellular cancer. J Clin Oncol, 5(10): 1566-1573.

Tang ZY, Liu KD, Bao YM, et al. 1990. Radioimmunotherapy in the multimodality treatment of hepatocellular carcinoma with reference to second-look resection. Cancer, 65: 211-215.

Yu YQ, Xu DB, Zhou XD, et al. 1993. Experience with liver resection after hepatic arterial chemoembolization for hepatocellular carcinoma. Cancer, 128: 224-226.

Zhang XH, Wu MC. 1989. Hepatic artery ligation and operative embolization. In: Tang ZY, Wu MC, Xia SS (eds), Primary liver cancer. Beijing: China Acad Publishers, Berlin: Springer-Verlag, 385-393.

樊嘉, 余业勤. 1995. 直径 12cm 以上原发性肝癌二期切除报告. 中国实用外科杂志, 15: 664, 665.

樊嘉, 余业勤, 吴志全, 等 .1997. 肝细胞癌经皮穿刺肝动脉化疗栓塞缩小后切除及疗效分析. 中华外科杂志, 35(12): 710-712.

陆继珍, 曹韵贞, 唐辰龙, 等. 1979. 原发性肝癌的选择性腹腔动脉和肝动脉造影 26 例分析. 上海医学, 2: 734-737.

陆继珍, 刘康达, 余业勤, 等. 1986. 人体肝细胞性肝癌血供的研究. 肿瘤, 6: 183-184.

陆继珍, 李炳鑫, 刘康达, 等. 1989. 超分割放疗与化疗交替方案治疗原发性肝癌的临床研究. 肿瘤, 9: 52-54.

马曾辰, 汤钊猷, 余业勤, 等. 1995. 原发性肝癌外科手术概念的更新和术后长期生存. 普外基础与临床杂志, 2 (1): 42-44.

汤钊猷, 余业勤, 周信达, 等. 1991. 不能切除肝癌的缩小疗法与序贯切除. 肿瘤,
　11: 145-147, 151.

余业勤, 汤钊猷, 周信达, 等. 1983. 大肝癌的分阶段治疗. 中华外科杂志,
　21(2): 92-93.

余业勤, 汤钊猷, 周信达. 1985. 术中肝动脉插管术技术的改进. 实用外科杂志,
　5: 5-7.

余业勤, 徐东波, 周信达, 等. 1991. 肝动脉化疗栓塞术后肝癌切除术 27 例分析.
　中国实用外科杂志, 11: 247-248.

周信达, 汤钊猷, 余业勤, 等. 1991. 肝动脉结扎和插管化疗治疗不能切除肝癌
　的评价. 中华外科杂志, 29(2): 87-89.

Part VII

Is Elevated Liver Enzymes in Liver Cancer a Surgical Contraindication?

The liver is an organ of the body with many important functions. It is also susceptible to various kinds of injury. The so called liver enzymes transaminases, especially ALT are actually not exclusively from the liver. The various forms of liver insult could be categorized as biologic, metabolic, traumatic or toxic. The fact that tumor growth could also be a form of insult has usually been ignored and neglected. In addition, we have seen many healthy teenagers being reported to have elevation of these enzymes, but without any evidence of liver disease. Their elevated enzyme level spontaneously returned to normal without any treatment. To date, the consensus is avoid surgery whenever liver enzymes are elevated. The fear is surgery might aggravate the injury and precipitate liver failure. Fulminant liver failure is highly lethal, not responding to any form of treatment, may be except liver transplantation. Elevated liver enzyme has been used as a biomarker to monitor progression of the injury. Actually, bilirubin is also a biomarker of liver disease. The phenomenon of "bilirubin-enzyme dissociation" should not be taken lightly. A high bilirubin not coupled with a similarly elevated enzyme level, but with a subnormal level is a dissociation. It is a bad omen and portends impending liver failure, signifying the hepatocyte has failed to respond to an insult and no enzyme is produced. After hepatectomy, the normal response is elevation of liver enzymes. The rise could be very high, at times even exceeding 2,000. However, it would return to normal during convalescence. This should be considered a physiologic response to stress without any pathologic sequelae like in hepatitis. Elevated enzyme per se should not be considered a surgical contraindication. When a liver cancer patient presents with an elevated enzyme level, the dilemma of "surgery or no surgery" is a live and death decision.

We encountered such a situation some years ago. After careful deliberation and exclusion of all possible etiologic factors for the rise in enzyme level, we boldly performed the resection. As expected, the elevation did not get worse but returned to normal. The patient is living and well with ongoing survival of 16 years. Subsequently, a similar case appeared and underwent surgery without any adverse effect. Ongoing survival was 12 years.

We strongly feel that such situations are not rare and deserve serious consideration. If we forget that tumor growth could also be the eliciting factor and blindly opted against surgery, the grave mistake would be like a judge setting a culprit free, but sentencing an innocent person a verdict of death, depriving his/her only chance of being salvaged. One has no right to take away the life of a person, be he/she healthy or sick. More cases and further in-depth studies are needed to validate our conception of indication breakthrough, as this might be applied to other malignancies as well.

Illustrative cases as follows.

Patient 1 (admission No. 389736)

Mr. XU had upper abdomen discomfort and a space-occupying lesion in the liver on B-US and MRI scanning. Although AFP was negative (4.6μg/L), liver cancer was highly suspected. Despite ALT elevated to 154U/L, without symptoms and signs of hepatitis, we decided to explore. In Jun 2002 at age 67 a 4.0cm×3.5cm×3.5cm cancer was located at the top of the right lobe of the liver with mild cirrhosis. A right partial hepatectomy was successfully performed and convalescence uneventful. In the absence of any special treatment, post-op ALT increased transient slightly, then gradually reverted to normal. Unfortunately, in Sep 2013, the 11th post-op year, his tumor recurred. A 1.8cm tumor was located in segment VII. He underwent a 2nd hepatectomy and recovered smoothly. The pathology reports of both operations were HCC. Follow-up by Jun 2015 at age 79, he was still alive and well with ongoing survival of 16 years.

Table 7.1 Perioperative ALT level

Date	ALT (U/L)	SB / SB' (μmol/L)
2012-6-1 before operation	154	31.1 / 11.3
2012-6-6 1st post-op day	235	34.3 / 14.2
2012-6-8 3rd post-op day	129	50.3 / 24.7
2012-6-10 5th post-op day	66	53.8 / 22.3
2012-6-13 8th post-op day	32	29 / 12.8
2012-6-19 14th post-op day	20	18.3 / 2.8

Patient 2 (admission No. 405198)

Mr. Wu had HBV infection 20 years ago. During hepatitis follow-up, he was found to have an elevated AFP and a space-occupying lesion in the liver. On B-US and CT，he had 2 resections for liver cancer. The first was performed in Mar 2003 at age 54. A 2.5cm tumor was located in the right lobe and a right partial hepatectomy was performed. After operation, AFP dropped from 573μg/L to normal. Two prophylactic TACEs were administered (Apr 2003 and Sep 2003). In May 2005, AFP elevated again and recurrence was suspected. Although treated again by 2 TACEs (May and Nov 2005), AFP did not turn negative and a new space-occupying lesion in the liver was found on B-US. A 2nd operation, left lateral hepatectomy was performed for a 2cm tumor in Feb 2006 at age 57. Convalescence was basically smooth. Pathology reports of both operations were HCC. Follow-up by May 2015 at age 67, he was still alive and well with ongoing survival of 12 years.

Before the 1st operation his ALT was normal (37U/L), but rose to exceed 2,000 post-op. Before the 2nd operation, ALT was elevated for 2 months and fluctuated between 157 U/L and 197U/L. There was no improvement with supportive treatment. Consent was obtained and we decided to operate. The patient's post-op ALT transient moderately rose further, then decreased to normal within two weeks.

Table 7.2   Perioperative ALT level during the 1st operation of patient

Date	ALT (U/L)	AST (U/L)	SB/ SB' (μmol/L)
2003-3-14 before operation	38	27	14.5 / 4.5
2003-3-20 1st post-op day	2431	2073	11.0/ 6.2
2003-3-24 5th post-op day	383	52	26.6 / 12.4
2003-3-27 8th post-op day	173	40	18.3 / 6.8

Table 7.3   Perioperative ALT level during the 2nd operation

Date	AFP (μg/L)	ALT (U/L)	AST(U/L) (g/L)	SB/SB' (μmol/L)	A/G
2006-2-7 before operation	1916.50	157	154	13.7 / 2.1	43 / 34
2006-2-9 1st post-op day	–	524	435	19.5 / 8.4	43 / 30
2006-2-11 3rd post-op day	–	447	154	55.7 / 19.0	51 / 29
2006-2-14 6th post-op day	–	155	42	37.4 / 16.9	38 / 27
2006-2-17 9th post-op day	355.80	75	32	22.7 / 11.7	39 / 33
2006-2-20 12th post-op day		55	35	18.9/11.2	30 / 35
2006-2-27 19th post-op day	61.52	46	46	16.8 / 4.7	34 / 41
2006-4-24 56th post-op day	6.04	53	–	9.8 / 4.4	36 / 35

As for ALT elevation before operation, we thought it was secondary to the TACE treatment. As the elevation did not return to normal with time and supportive treatment, we decided to explore. Surgery confirmed that recurrent cancer was the culprit for the elevation. Our experience is no matter what caused the ALT elevation, it per se does not mean there is serious liver damage and contraindicated operation.

ALT is a sensitive indicator of liver injury, but bilirubin is the most important one. The so-called "bilirubin-enzyme dissociation" phenomenon portends irreversible hepatic damage. Our clinical practice validated that ALT elevated 3 or 4 times normal, or even higher before hepatectomy, did not affect safety of hepatic surgery. When ALT increased to 10, or even 50 times normal after operation, as long as bilirubin does not increase abnormally, normal liver function could be restored. In "bilirubin-enzyme dissociation" subnormal ALT is of great value in predicting liver failure.

A more vivid metaphor is that, when a child cried aloud after an accident, there might not be any problem of significant concern. However, if the child remained quiet, possibly quite serious damage had occurred like in "bilirubin-enzyme dissociation" (high bilirubin, low ALT), perhaps danger is ahead.

Of course, we do not blindly ignore ALT elevation. Instead, we carry out a comprehensive examination to exclude other conditions that could cause the elevation. After weighing advantages and disadvantages, we should perform hepatectomy timely after obtaining the patient's understanding and consent to yield the best effect.

References

马曾辰, 方涛林, 孙惠川, 等. 2002. 血友病患者的肝癌切除治疗. 中国临床医学, 9 (2): 124-126.

马曾辰. 2016. 不要被转氨酶升高吓倒, 为部分伴转氨酶升高肝癌患者开手术绿灯. 见: 马曾辰. 突破: 88 例肝癌患者手术后 20—48 年长期生存. 北京: 科学出版社, 163-166.

周信达, 汤钊猷, 余业勤. 1980. 原发性肝癌手术切除后肝功能变化及其处理. 中华医学杂志, 60(10): 606-611.

Part VIII

Challenges and Our Preliminary Efforts

It is well known that cancer of the liver is a dreadful disease. It is highly malignant, prone to recur and metastasize, clinical course short, prognosis poor and mortality high. Once diagnosed, further lifespan can only be counted in months. Faced with this gloomy situation, physicians in China accepted the challenge to tackle this tough nut as of the 1950s. We tried all forms of treatment. As experience cumulated, this obsolete pessimistic view has been replaced by an optimistic one. We found that this cancer could be detected early and the biocharacter of some were not that malignant as formerly believed. Furthermore, a patient's will to live and anticancer determination were not that frail. Surgery and other treatments were safe and often very effective. In short, part of liver cancer could be treated and lifespan counted in years instead of months. In fact, some even achieved long-term survival with good quality of life to reach a ripe old age.

Advance in clinical research of liver cancer is mostly centered around therapeutic results. To improve these results, the key is "renew our knowledge of this disease". Liver cancer is a systemic as well as local disease with variable malignancy. Recurrence and metastasis are prone but not dead set adverse qualities. All these make surgical resection and other forms of local treatment become rational.

The following are gems to take home:

(1) Surgical resection is the mainstay and most important form of treatment for improved results, especially for long-term survival. Thoroughness is the most important value of resection. The number of patients treated without surgical resection far exceeded those subjected to resection, but few achieved long-term survival. On the other hand, among the long-term survivors, over 90% were treated by surgical resection. Therefore, to improve results the key is resection or resection supplemented with other modalities of comprehensive treatment. Naturally, early diagnosis and means to improve early diagnosis should not be neglected. If research is not on what is important, but set on a

wrong path, a good harvest can rarely be achieved and efforts wasted. Though local treatments also can be highly tumorcidal, indications are limited and cannot replace surgical resection. Technical advances coupled with cumulated experiences, the safety of surgery has been greatly enhanced. In the hands of an experienced surgeon, the surgical mortality is less than 1%. Though surgery is a form of trauma, convalescence is usually rapid and uneventful. Quality of life is like that of any other healthy person. The most heartening part is certain patients will have long-term survival and lifespan unaffected.

(2) There is no standardized mode of resection for liver cancer. We feel irregular resection should be the main form for liver cancer. The anatomic or regular resection sacrifices too much normal liver parenchyma unnecessarily. Our irregular resection has achieved very good results, being equally radical with long-term survival. We don't advocate segmentectomy as it lacks thoroughness. Cancer does not limit its growth just within a segment. One need not worry about blood supply to the remaining liver after an irregular resection. The liver is richly supplied. Purpose of an irregular resection is to spare as much normal liver tissue as possible, especially in a right half liver cancer. On the other hand, we are not entirely against anatomic hepatectomy. If the right side cancer is exceptionally large or located at the middle of the lobe, we still feel a right hemihepatectomy (anatomic resection) would be the best option. For those on the left side, as the left liver is much smaller, anatomic or regular resection does not sacrifice undue amounts of normal liver tissue. A left lateral lobectomy and left hemihepatectomy are acceptable procedures. Our indications are "left regular and right irregular" to allow option be more flexible.

(3) Resection of liver cancer still needs to strictly follow the basic principles of tumor surgery, the "nontouch principle" Resection is usually more difficult than with other tumors. But difficulty does not mean that one can ignore the nontouch principle. We usually insert sutures on both sides of the contemplated incision for traction on normal liver tissue to avoid direct contact with the tumor. Direct

tumor manipulation would inevitably lead to spread from pressure of the squeezing. The incision should be sufficiently adequate to permit facilitation of the procedure and all perihepatic ligaments fully mobilized. Radical resection of liver cancer differs from other tumors is that for HCC there is no need to clear hilum lymph nodes. A set safety resection margin is not practical in liver surgery and carries too much risk. However, the tumor must be completely resected. If possible, a 1cm or more margin can be considered.

Safety should never be neglected. Blood loss is an important issue. Excess blood loss is not only lethal, it also affects recovery and quality of life. Too many blood transfusions can bring about other adverse effects. Our dogma is "conserve every drop of blood and control its loss to a minimum". We advocate application of the Pringle maneuver to minimize blood loss. We strongly oppose the concept of "trade ischemia for blood loss". In our experience of thousands of hepatectomies, we have not yet witnessed liver failure due to transient occlusion of the hilum. On the other hand, excessive blood loss or forced passive hilum occlusion led to serious consequences. Occlusion period and repeated times vary with degree of cirrhosis and magnitude of the resection. Occlusion period is usually 5–10min with an interval of 3–5min free flow before the next occlusion. In the hands of an experienced surgeon, a limited magnitude resection can be completed without the need of occlusion. Old age and cirrhosis are not surgical contraindications, but do increase risks. In such cases, indications for surgery should be more stringent, magnitude of the procedure as well as operative time be limited and minimize blood loss. A green surgeon should not mistakenly feel that a small cancer because of its size is an easy highly safe procedure. In fact, many cancers are small because cirrhosis limited their expansion, risks are higher and surgical mortality is not rare.

(4) There are 2 views on cancer recurrence. One is that it is considered a late stage phenomenon and opted against further surgery. The other is more aggressive, opted for resection if conditions permit. We are of the opinion that if the recurrence is solitary or extent limited,

resection is indicated. A patient's vitality and reserve are surprisingly abundant, can easily accommodate the stress and trauma of a second and even a third resection. Our belief is further strengthened by the results of such resections. Convalescence is smooth and final result ideal. Of course, the added surgery is for cure and not palliation. In addition, other local treatments as supplement can also be considered if needed.

Similarly, we are also very aggressive with metastasis. The most frequent site is the lungs. When solitary or multiple but close together, we also advocate resection. This is because we already have quite a number of successive cases to support our stand. Cases 8, 10, 12 and 28 in our series all had resection of their pulmonary metastasis and survived over 20 years. Our aggressive attitude is based on our practical experience. We hope more colleagues with more successive cases will eventually replace the obsolete antiquated pessimistic textbook view to the benefit of more patients.

(5) The liver has 2 sets of blood supply, different from other organs. They are the hepatic artery and portal vein. Hepatocytes derive nutrients almost fully from the portal vein. Once the portal vein supply is cut off the liver cannot survive. The hepatic artery only plays a minor role in nutrient supply. Clinically, it has been confirmed that cut off of the arterial supply does not lead to necrosis of the liver. Hence, in case of bleeding from the liver ligation of the hepatic artery will control the bleeding but not induce necrosis of the liver.

It has been proven that HCC derives its blood supply mainly from the hepatic artery. Occlusion of the artery will inhibit growth and vitality of cancer cells. Based on this finding, we can tie off the artery to treat HCC. Clinically, ligation of the hepatic artery led to decreased vitality and apoptosis of the cancer cells. Imaging studies showed decreased intratumor blood flow, tumor necrosis and reduction of tumor size. The patient's condition improved significantly and lifespan extended. The procedure did not cause death of normal liver tissue or impaired liver function. Artery ligation is often combined with cannulation, followed by intermittent infusion chemotherapy for the cancer. Such treatment is superior to that of only ligation or only cannulation. The basis is the same in percutaneous hepatic artery interventional treatment. The latter's advantage is that open surgery is avoided, but the tumorcidal effect is less satisfactory, not as complete or thorough as with open surgery.

(6) HCC maybe early or late and size small or large. When a cancer is too large or too late not suitable for resection, the 2-step resection comes to the fore. The pre-requisite is that after the 1st-step treatment, the cancer is reduced in size or general condition improved. In our experience, the effects of hepatic artery surgery are most prominent and part of patients become suitable to accept the 2nd-step treatment. If the large tumor had reduced in size, became further away from major vessels, remaining normal liver adequate to support life and probable cure possible, then the 2nd-step treatment could be considered. We feel conservative treatment of liver cancer is rarely successful, while the odds are much improved if we can complete the 2nd-step resection. Many patients made full use of this chance and achieved long-term survival. Case 22 accepted the 2-step resection 35 years ago and on follow-up by Sep 2015, he was still alive and well. .

(7) HCC differs from other solid tumors. It has a tendency to invade blood vessels and bile ducts to form tumor thrombi. This signifies that the tumor is highly invasive and the disease is progressing. Liver cancer thrombi can be divided according to their location. They are portal vein, bile duct, hepatic vein and inferior vena cava tumor thrombi. The last one is an extension from the hepatic vein or short hepatic vein. Based on its magnitude, the thrombus can be in the main trunk or a branch. We should not be pessimistic regarding treatment and prognosis of the tumor thrombus. When a thrombus can be resected En Bloc with the tumor, we should not hesitate to do so. For example, in a left lateral lobectomy the left hepatic vein tumor thrombus can be removed at the same time. In left hemihepatectomy, the left portal vein or left bile duct together with the tumor thrombus should also be removed. Likewise, this is the same with a right hemihepatectomy. Our experience dated back to 40 years ago, case 8 a large left lateral lobe liver cancer with a left hepatic vein tumor thrombus was subjected to a left lateral lobectomy and removal of the thrombus. The patient survived 32 years but eventually died of liver cirrhosis. There are many successful cases. We feel surgical indication should be appropriate. Regarding a tumor thrombus, we should not be blindly pessimistic. We are also against palliative partial resection of the tumor and thrombus, the so called tumor mass reduction procedure.

(8) We should have better understanding of the liver enzyme and surgical treatment of liver cancer. ALT can be a representative of the liver enzymes. Hepatologists have long ago defined enzyme elevation could be physiologic or pathologic. Growth development in an adolescent and violent exercise could cause elevation of liver enzymes. As hepatic surgeons, we should have an even more in-depth understanding. After hepatectomy, ALT elevation is a normal response. The elevation is variable and transient. It could reach to over 2,000U/ L but return to normal in a few days. This physiologic elevation has no relation whatsoever with the course of convalescence or outcome. In our experience, such elevation is not to be feared. On the other hand, "bilirubin-enzyme dissociation" and misinterpretation of the elevation are more fearful. Consequence of the latter would be delayed or loss of the optimal time for treatment. If the physiologic elevation in a liver cancer patient is mistaken to be pathologic due to hepatitis and opted against surgery for fear of aggravating the hepatitis, delaying surgery until the elevation returned normal, the consequence and outcome should be quite obvious.

Fortunately, we timely corrected the above misconception and timely operated on the cancer patient with a physiologic elevation and salvaged the patient, who also became a long-term survivor. We have met with two classical cases of liver cancer with elevated ALT. Their respective survivals are 13 and 12 years, both living and well. Details have already been given elsewhere in this text. We feel tumor growth can also induce enzyme elevation and only resection of the tumor can make the elevation return to normal. If surgery is delayed until ALT has returned to normal the outcome is self evident.

Similar not classical cases are not rare. Treatment of liver cancer should never be delayed. A patient (Admission No. 375928) had coexisting hemophilia. After consultation with Hematology specialists and balancing risks, the patient was given large amounts of factor Ⅷ and operated on under close monitoring. The patient recovered uneventfully.

Improved treatment results, especially long-term results do not depend on sophisticated equipment and advanced skills or technique. The only determining factor is complete understanding of the disease and a scientific mind.

(9) In the 1960s, the few liver cancer patients with a symptomatic mass were benefited by the development of liver surgery. In the 1970s, part of liver cancer patients was saved by the discovery of Alpha-fetoprotein (AFP) and its clinical application. From the end of the 1970s to the early 1980s, imaging equipment (B-US, CT, MRI, etc) made their debut and outcome of liver cancer greatly improved. Imaging studies could supplement the shortcomings of AFP in the diagnosis of liver cancer. They could accurately detect as well as locate the cancer are their merits. A tumor 1cm in size could clearly be visualized. The intrahepatic tubular structures are well delineated. All these contributed to the successful application of liver surgery and local treatments. We feel that B-US has the merits of being simple, efficient, accurate and nontraumatic, should be treated as valuable as CT and MRI. In fact, they are complementary tools. CT and MRI become most important in AFP negative situations. Experience accumulated with these measures can make diagnosis of most liver cancers without fail. It is no longer necessary to perform needle biopsy as a routine for diagnosis.

Improved treatment outcome depends on treatment as well as diagnosis. In other words, it depends on advances in science and technology and more importantly on continuously being renewed basic concepts. In the past, we felt AFP less than 200μg/L was not cancer. Arbitrarily, the diagnostic criterion was set at greater than 400μg/L persistent for 4 weeks or greater than 200μg/L persistent for 8 weeks. With time and as experience cumulated, we found that 18% of cancer patients had low elevated AFP (21-200μg/L). Our present revised view is that AFP could be high, low level high or even normal. With this renewed AFP concept, there would be less missed diagnosis and more timely treatment. Furthermore, after resection of an AFP positive cancer the elevated AFP would gradually return to normal. It is a useful tool in monitoring progression of the disease as well as alert recurrence and metastasis. With recurrence, AFP could be elevated or even become negative. A positive patient after resection should not only monitor AFP regularly. Imaging studies are equally important to minimize missed diagnosis because of possible change in biocharacter of the cancer. AFP positive becomes negative and can only be detected by imaging studies. Similarly, in a negative patient with recurrence AFP might not continue to remain negative. Neglected regular monitoring would miss a recurrence that happened to have changed to become positive. Never forget that timely detection means timely treatment and a more favorable outcome.

(10) As experience cumulated with time, advances in science and treatment of cancer improved. Liver cancer patients are no longer contend with short-term survival of 1-5 years. Their goal is at least 10 years long-term survival with good quality of life. Actually, quite a number of patients have already realized this goal. We feel liver cancer research in the future should center around the goal of long-term survival. So called long-term is at least 10 years. Short-term is 1-5 years and mid-long-term 5-10 years.

Liver surgery was established in the 1960s in China. As of the 1980s, quite a number of over 10 years survival liver cancer patients after treatment have been reported. The longest survival was 48 years (case 2) and the oldest survivor reached 99 years of age (case 12). After half a century, how can we still be satisfied with the survival goal of

1, 3 and 5 years. We are too much behind time, far from the wish of patients and in no position to realize the dreams of patients. To make their dreams come true, we need to switch place with patients, discard our obsolete conception, try to think as they do and work for the goal of long-term survival. If a patient were 35 years old, 5-year survival would mean the patient could live to 40, which is much too subpar the normal life expectancy of the 21st century. How could the patient be contend. As healers of the sick, we should be ashamed of our "not doing" and efforts wasted on the wrong path.

To date, surgery for liver cancer is already well established. In the absence of satisfactory chemotherapeutic agents, surgical resection is still the most effective treatment. Local treatments (cryotherapy, microwave, radiofrequency ablation, intratumor ethanol injection, etc) and percutaneous hepatic artery interventional procedures are also tumorcidal. Though their effect are less satisfactory than surgical resection, can still be considered. In fact, open hepatic artery ligation with cannulation followed by infusion chemotherapy has quite good effects. If the above measures either used alone or comprehensively will push the patient another step further towards long-term survival and the joy of long life.

The treatment of liver cancer should not be taken as a single treatment is enough. It actually is a systematic project that at times involves repeated or repeated comprehensive treatments. Hence, clinicians should, with a patient as the receiving center, dispense the most effective and appropriate treatment. Despite hardship and tedious work, we should insist on data documentation, follow-ups, revisits and a positive aggressive attitude regarding recurrence/metastasis. Only thus can we achieve good results to satisfy our patients.

As recurrence could occur decades later (case 1), follow-up for life should be emphasized and never give-up even when recurrence occurs repeatedly. With timely follow-up and prompt appropriate treatment, salvage might still be achieved. Of course, the benefits and risks of any treatment should be weighed carefully prior to being carried out. Safety of the patient should be our only goal. If more than one morbidity coexist, the most lethal or life threatening one should have the treatment priority with the others priority timed in order of importance. Furthermore, never forget to learn from our setbacks to avoid repeating the same mistakes.

References

Bismuth H, Houssin D, Castaing, et al. 1982. Major and minor segmentectomies "reglees" in liver surgery. World J Surg, 6(1): 10-24.

Lawrence GH, Grauman D, Lasersohn, et al. 1966. Primary carcinoma of the liver. Amer J Surg, 112(2): 200-210.

Starzl TE, Koep LJ, Weid R III, et al. 1980. Right trisegmentectomy for hepatic neoplasms. Surg Gynecol Obstet, 150(2): 208-214.

Thompson HH, Tompkins RK, Longmire WP. 1983. Major hepatic resection: a 25-year experience. Ann Surg, 197(4): 375-388.

Yu YQ, Xu DB, Zhou XD, et al. 1993. Experience with liver resection after hepatic arterial chemoembolization for hepatocellular carcinoma. Cancer, 128: 224-226.

李家忠, 叶宗典, 卢运侃, 黄萃庭, 曾宪九. 1959. 广泛肝叶切除术-附16例报告. 中华外科杂志, 7(12): 1151-1159.

马曾辰, 吴肇光, 汤钊猷. 2008. 肝癌生存43年一例. 中华肿瘤杂志, 30(3): 210.

孙益红, 秦新裕, 汪学非, 等. 2003. 胃癌肝转移的手术治疗. 中华胃肠外科杂志, 6(5): 301-304.

余业勤, 汤钊猷, 周信达. 1978. 切除小肝癌的经验. 中华外科杂志, 16(5): 266-268.

Acknowledgement

To date, report of long-term survival in liver cancer has been few and not systematically in detail or in large numbers. The staff of the Liver Cancer Institute at Zhong Shan Hospital has taken up this task as an important project in their work. The manpower involved is immense, tremendous and consists of surgeons and internists, as well as TCM practitioners. To name a few, internists included peers that analyzed clinical manifestations and those that championed screening to detect early cancer. Professor Zhaoyou Tang, Founder of the Liver Cancer Institute and Member of the Chinese Academy of Engineering first pointed out small cancers do not need regular hepatectomy and irregular resection yielded equally good results. The advent of liver transplantation might become an established mode of treatment in the future.

This volume on long-term survival in liver cancer is small in size, but its contents full of gems. It is not the work of a single center. Investigators in China and from around the world have gratefully shared their work to elucidate many aspects of liver cancer. Their contributions are equally important, so are the many surgical fellows and young clinicians in training at Zhong Shan Hospital. Confronted with the heavy workload, we deeply thank this strong force of manpower and cooperation of the patients that made completion of this monogram in time possible.

Our special thanks and deepest gratitude must go to Professor Zhaoguang Wu, who initiated resection of liver cancer at Zhong Shan Hospital and broke through the 40-year survival mark to strengthen our belief that long-term survival in liver cancer could be realized. We cannot adequately express how much we have enjoyed his wit, wisdom and good fellowship. Most of the uniformity and clarity of expression are due to his artistic sense of the English language and his inciseful clarity of thought.

We also wish to thank our families for allowing us to pitch whole heartedly in piling data for this monogram by relieving our duties at home.

The fact that this monogram will appear within less than 24 months after conception is due largely to the grace and staunch support of Ms Xiaoling Yang of the Science Press. Her efforts facilitated and expedited publication of this monogram.

Index